# IT CAN (AND DOES) HAPPEN HERE!

## ONE PHYSICIAN'S FOUR DECADES-LONG JOURNEY AS CORONER IN RURAL NORTH IDAHO

### ROBERT S. WEST, MD, FACS

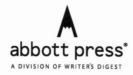

abbott press®

A DIVISION OF WRITER'S DIGEST

Abbott Press books may be ordered through booksellers or by contacting:

Abbott Press
1663 Liberty Drive
Bloomington, IN 47403
www.abbottpress.com
Phone: 1-866-697-5310

Because of the dynamic nature of the Internet, any web addresses or links contained in
this book may have changed since publication and may no longer be valid. The views
expressed in this work are solely those of the author and do not necessarily reflect the
views of the publisher, and the publisher hereby disclaims any responsibility for them.

Any people depicted in stock imagery provided by Thinkstock are models,
and such images are being used for illustrative purposes only.
Certain stock imagery © Thinkstock.

ISBN: 978-1-4582-1544-4 (sc)
ISBN: 978-1-4582-1543-7 (hc)
ISBN: 978-1-4582-1542-0 (e)

Library of Congress Control Number: 2014906841

Printed in the United States of America.

Abbott Press rev. date: 04/29/2014

# CONTENTS

# PREFACE

My purpose for writing this book is to trace the history and development of the Coroner/Medical Examiner system (or non-system) in the United States and, in particular, Idaho. The first Medical Examiner system was established in Boston in 1877. The appointment of Dr. Charles Norris as the New York Medical Examiner in 1890 and, later, the addition of toxicologist Alexander Gettler, PhD heralded the establishment of a true forensic examiner system which set the standard for many years.[1]

I am not implying that the cases described represent the general run of cases, only to describe unusual incidents requiring specific knowledge, attention to detail, and which call on many resources to reach conclusions about the cause and manner of death. I found it professionally challenging and gratifying to serve the citizens of Kootenai County. I hope that the reader will find the book interesting and insightful.

A note of caution: Some descriptions and photos in this book are graphic and readers may find them disturbing. The book may not be suitable for younger readers. Parental discretion is advised. All incidents reflect my perception of events occurring during my tenure as the Kootenai County Deputy Coroner from 1970 to1984, and Coroner from 1984 until 2011. Pseudonyms have been used to protect the identities of private individuals and victims. Public officials and entities are identified by name.

---

[1]   "Charles Norris (1868-1935) and Thomas A. Gonzales (1878-1956) New York's Forensic Pioneers" American Journal of Forensic Medical Pathology 1987 Dec. 8 (4) pp 350-353

# Foreword

*It Can (And Does) Happen Here* illustrates precisely why the current coroner/medical examiner system needs and deserves improvement.

Dr. West draws on four decades of death investigation in rural Kootenai County, Idaho. From "routine" unattended deaths to complex murders to horrific accidents, rural coroners are expected to determine the cause and manner of death with the same accuracy and precision as urban forensic facilities.

As in many jurisdictions, Idaho has minimal requisite qualifications for the coroner. This book addresses the ignorance and apathy the public has about the realities of our current system (or as he refers to it, our *non*system.)

He draws on a wealth of experience to focus on the pathos and sometimes puzzling aspects of the position of coroner. The occasional unexpected findings and reflection on the vagaries of the human condition are presented well.

This is an intense and absorbing read which will challenge you to become active in your community to bring about the changes he suggests.

Martha W. Hopkins

# CHAPTER 1

# SYSTEM OR
# NON-SYSTEM

*The strobe lights of multiple squad cars flashed over the neighborhood on a February night in 1986. Dr. Bob West, a general surgeon and the Kootenai County Coroner—stopped at the mobile command post on Fourteenth Street in Coeur d'Alene, Idaho. He contacted the Special Weapons and Tactics (SWAT) team commander to get a briefing on the incident.*

*"We have a twenty-eight-year-old 'psycho' holed up in this house, threatening to kill anyone who tries to enter. The windows and doors are barricaded, the phone lines have been cut, and several shots have been fired. There has been no sign of activity in the house for the past thirty minutes and the chief of police requested the coroner and paramedics to be on scene.*

*"We do not know much else about him. The family reports a marked change in his personality over the past six months. He has become moody, withdrawn, and very paranoid and has complained of severe headaches. Kootenai County Sheriff deputies have responded to the home several times for domestic violence issues. They say he was an electrician for a local contracting firm and always been a safety-conscious worker."*

*SWAT team members had the house surrounded and hailed the occupant to come out. Hearing no response, they forced the lock on the front door, entered the house, and found the victim with a gunshot wound to the head. A revolver lay next to the victim with a single spent cartridge in the chamber. The paramedics on scene confirmed the death and returned*

1

to quarters. *The lead detective from the sheriff's office began a systematic scene investigation, taking photos of the victim, the weapon, and the interior of the house.*

*After the investigators completed their initial investigation, Dr. West and the on-call funeral home personnel entered the home to remove the victim. The detective asked whether there would be an autopsy. It seemed clear the victim had committed suicide. Even though the case seemed straightforward, Dr. West explained that there would be a full autopsy, including toxicology, conducted by the Spokane County Medical Examiner's (SCME) office.*

*Further investigation revealed that six months previously, while working as an electrician at the Coeur d'Alene Resort Golf Course's signature floating fourteenth green, the victim was working in the mechanical equipment room. Mercury switches in that room operate pumps to ensure the green stays level. As the green shifts side to side, or fore and aft, the switches activate pumps, which force water into ballast tanks, keeping the green's surface level.*

*As the victim was working on the electrical system, one of the mercury switches exploded, vaporizing the mercury and the victim inhaled the poisonous mercuric oxide fumes. The room was subsequently ventilated. The electricians were not evaluated by physicians.*

*The victim's toxicology from the autopsy results came back showing marked elevation of serum mercury levels. Further testing showed the effects of chronic mercury poisoning as the likely cause of deterioration in mental status of the victim.*

This would explain the "mad hatter syndrome" symptoms in the victim. Long before Louis Carroll penned *Alice in Wonderland*, workers in hat factories used mercury compounds while working felt for hats. They experienced headaches, anemia, and personality changes and eventually became demented, hence, the name "mad hatter."

This case was an industrial accident, *not* a suicide. The subsequent wrongful death lawsuit did not make the coroner any friends in the resort's management. However, it did illustrate the type of investigation necessary, even in rural Idaho.

It also demonstrates the need for coroners to make their own investigation in each case and gather the information from both the autopsy and toxicology. The elevated blood mercury levels were not expected in this case. Coroners must educate themselves of the effects of various toxins, mercury in this case, but also a variety of substances seen in other cases.

*   *   *

The term *coroner* dates back to medieval England. The Magna Carta, signed at Runnymede in 1215, states: "...No sheriff, constable, *coroners,* or others of our bailiffs shall hold pleas of our crown." At that time, one of the duties of the coroner was to collect fees owed to the crown from the estate or family of deceased persons.

In the United States, as the persons responsible for creating and signing death certificates and burial permits evolved into the present system, there have been wide-ranging abuses and less-than-professional practices. In New York City in 1866, burial permits were sold to murderers to bury their victims. Twelve percent of physicians responsible for completing and signing death certificates have *no* training in correctly listing the cause and manner of death. The error rates on death certificates range up to 29 percent. There continues to be reluctance to list socially unacceptable causes and/or manner of death (e.g., syphilis, alcoholism, alcoholic cirrhosis, HIV/AIDs, suicide, homicide, or accidental deaths). When law enforcement shoots a person in the process of apprehension, the manner of death is homicide. The review panel and prosecutor make the determination as to justification or not. It is not uncommon for the coroner's office to receive inquiries as to why these cases are considered a homicide.

The National Academy of Science report, "Strengthening Forensic Science in the United States: A Path Forward,"[2] gives a detailed overview of the problem and suggested paths for resolving the deficiencies.

---

[2]   *Strengthening Forensic Science in the United States"* National Academies Press, 2009

The general public frequently misunderstands several of the terms listed below:

1. **Medical examiner:** A licensed physician (MD or DO) who has completed a pathology residency, a fellowship in forensic pathology and is certified in both pathology and forensic pathology by the American Board of Pathology.

2. **Physician coroner:** A physician (MD or DO) who has graduated from medical school and is licensed to practice medicine. He/she may or may not have had post-graduate training in death investigation.

3. **Death investigator:** A person who has completed one or more courses in death investigation. These may be sponsored by universities, hospitals, and/or state coroner organizations. Many national and state organizations offer certification as a death investigator.

4. **Nurse coroner:** A nurse (RN or LPN) who graduated from a nursing program and is licensed to practice as a nurse. He/she may or may not have trained in death investigation.

5. **Mortician or funeral home technician coroner:** A funeral home employee trained in the procedures involved in the removal, embalming, and care of deceased persons. He/she may or may not have trained in death investigation.

6. **Coroner:** Any of the above persons elected, appointed, or otherwise qualified for the position as specified in the state code. Recent changes in the Idaho code have added periodic coroner continuing education requirements for coroners.

This list, while not exhaustive, illustrates the wide range of persons who comprise the coroner/medical examiner system in the United States.

## My Background

This was the status of the coroner/medical examiner system when Dr. William T. Wood, Kootenai County Coroner, called me in July 1970 to ask if I would cover coroner calls while he was at the Idaho Medical Association meeting in Sun Valley. Since statehood in 1890, local physicians had acted as coroner in Kootenai County as a part of their responsibility to the public. The Idaho code states, "The coroner shall be twenty-one years of age and a resident of the county for one year."[3]

I asked him what my duties were. His response: "Raise your right hand." With a few words, I became a deputy coroner for Kootenai County, with the duty and legal responsibility to investigate all deaths by "other than natural causes" within the 1,441 square miles of Kootenai County.

He also failed to inform me, "The coroner shall act as sheriff in the event of the death, arrest, or other incapacitation of the sheriff."[4]

While this was daunting to a young surgeon recently arrived to Coeur d'Alene, I did have some background in death investigation.

As a freshman at the University of North Dakota Medical School Gross Anatomy Lab, my partner and I found an impacted piece of steak in the posterior pharynx of our cadaver. Our "patient" had died of a "café coronary" long before Dr. Heimlich described his eponymic maneuver.

Later, at Harvard Medical School, students attended a weekly death conference where the Suffolk County (Boston) Medical Examiner would detail the many complex cases presented to his office.

Boston was still reeling from the disastrous Cocoanut Grove fire of November 28, 1942, which resulted in 492 deaths. Most of these deaths were caused by smoke inhalation. One good result from that tragedy: public buildings afterward were required to have self-contained emergency lighting and unlocked exits.

---

3    Idaho Code: Chapter 34, Sec. 6422 (Qualifications for Coroner)
4    Idaho Code: Chapter 31, Sec. 2801-2807 (Coroner to act as Sheriff)

We were required to attend all autopsies while on the surgical service of the Massachusetts General and Beth Israel Hospitals.

After a rotating internship at Chelsea Naval Hospital in the United States Navy Medical Corps, I served at the US Naval Station Hospital, Argentia, Newfoundland. We had no pathologist on staff. We transported our autopsy cases eighty miles to and from St. Johns, Newfoundland. Occasionally US Coast Guard Cutters would dock at Argentia with the body of a crewman who had succumbed to the frigid waters of the North Atlantic during their thirty-day patrols at Ocean Station Charlie. These cases were airlifted stateside to appropriate facilities.

*An Irish physician assigned to a British submarine which docked at Argentia over St. Patrick's Day managed to drive a borrowed car off the harbor dock at two o'clock in the morning. We found his body clinging to a piling less than three feet below the surface. The Royal Navy arranged for his removal to England.*

Noncombat military death statistics reflect alcohol's impact on more than 50 percent of motor vehicle deaths. Infrequently, flight crews would break the "five hours from bottle to throttle" rule. An F-4 Phantom Jet pilot drowned in an Officer's Club swimming pool after flying from Virginia to the Jacksonville Naval Air Station with less that two hours sleep in the previous forty-eight hours.

I witnessed the effects of alcohol in many deaths while serving as a surgical resident at the University of Vermont Medical Center Hospitals. I also performed several autopsies under supervision while on a pathology rotation to determine the cause of death. This included reviewing the medical records, laboratory and X-ray results, the microscopic slides, and then writing the final report detailing the cause of death.

I attended a mass-casualty management course at Brooke Army Medical Center, Fort Sam Houston, San Antonio, Texas, where mock-up casualties were triaged under battlefield conditions. I spent a week at the Armed Forces Institute of Pathology reviewing various cases from its vast collection and attending clinico-pathological conferences.

Nevertheless, I never considered myself a pathologist (or a forensic pathologist.) Rather, these experiences contributed to my basic fund of knowledge.

# Kootenai County Coroner History

The lake city of Coeur d'Alene, where I have resided since 1969, is thirty miles across the border from Spokane, Washington. The Idaho Panhandle is bisected by Interstate 90 and U.S. 95 and surrounded by a million acres of the Panhandle National Forest. The area's five lumber mills, the Silver Valley Mines, and the Kaiser Aluminum Rolling Mill in the Spokane Valley resulted in a steady stream of industrial accidents.

Tourists have flocked to the lakes and streams of North Idaho since the 1920s. During World War II, the Farragut Naval Training facility on Lake Pend Oreille provided sailors on liberty a good time in the bars and dance halls of the Lake City. Canadians with lake homes vacationed here in large numbers.

Kootenai County has had many physician-coroners since statehood. It was considered a part of a physician's civic duty. In Idaho, the Coroner is an elected, partisan position with a four-year term. Most Idaho Coroners are not physicians. There were only three physician-coroners in the State of Idaho between 1984 and 2010.

As of this writing, the non-physician coroners of Ada, Canyon, Twin Falls, and Bannock counties employ forensic pathologists who also provide forensic services to adjacent counties. The Spokane County Medical Examiner's (SCME) office also provides forensic services for the five northern Idaho counties. These positions are presently held by: two nurse-coroners, and three mortician-coroners.

Contract forensic pathologists provide forensic services to other counties on rare occasions such as a private request for an autopsy or for a "second opinion" autopsy. These cases are paid for by the requester.

Nationally, there is great misunderstanding of the dichotomy between the public's perception and the realities of this hodge-podge Coroner/Medical Examiner "non-system." The public assumes *all* coroners are board-certified Medical Examiners with the training, facilities and expertise to produce uniformly accurate results in one hour or less, as seen on the TV program *CSI Miami*. The 2011 NOVA public television documentary *Post-Mortem* chronicled a dismal picture of some of the worst deficiencies of the current coroner-medical examiner system. State and local funding entities do *not* come close to supporting the type of forensic systems necessary to provide even basic functions. Many coroners are not prepared to investigate coroner cases personally and on-scene regardless of the circumstances, distance, or time of day.

Professionally, there are few incentives to attract physicians or other persons to the field. Careers in forensic medicine are not encouraged by college pre-medical counselors. Medical students and pathology residents are seldom encouraged to enter this field of medicine. The financial rewards pale in comparison to the more lucrative specialties. A forensic pathologist typically spends thirteen to fifteen years of post-secondary education and may acquire $150,000–200,000 of student loan debt before reaching his/her first position as a medical examiner.

Much of this will have to change before we begin to address the current shortfall of some 1,500 qualified medical examiners in the United States Many current medical examiners are approaching retirement age. The lack of new physicians entering the training pipeline ensures that the problem will persist or worsen in the future.

One of the frequent comments heard from those who prefer to maintain the status quo of this system is: "Why do you need such an expensive, complex system? Nothing ever happens *here* like it does in New York or Los Angeles." or "We just need an Idaho coroner to complete the death certificates and authorize cremations." My answer to that is: "It *can* and *does* happen here!" Coupled with the above is the public's aversion to the whole subject of death and dying. Even physicians attending inpatients at Kootenai Medical Center (KMC) occasionally decline to sign death certificates, even though they were the attending on the case for several days in the intensive care unit. When death certificates default to the coroner for signature, families question as to why the coroner was involved.

I hope the following chapters will document my experiences and recognize the efforts of coroners in Idaho and other jurisdictions who carry out their duties in the face of apathy, ignorance and false conservatism.

We seldom address the issue of death in an open manner. The public and even my medical colleagues would occasionally comment to patients "...do you really *want* the coroner to be your surgeon?" My fellow elected county officers trailed my vote tally in several successive election cycles. However, the coroner's budget still comprises less than 1 percent of the total county budget.

Of course, none of the limitations above are operative when it is *your* child, spouse or other relative who is a murder victim, or dies in some bizarre manner. You want every resource utilized to bring perpetrators to justice and to exonerate the innocent.

My experience has been that the vast majority of coroners and medical examiners are extremely professional and diligent in performing their duties. They operate with scant resources in remote communities, and face the scrutiny of the public, law enforcement and the justice system. They must exhibit professional standards equivalent to the most advanced forensic medical examiner's office. All coroners must have a smooth working relationship with law enforcement, funeral homes, the public, and the media.

I hope this book will inspire the kind of financial and community support necessary to improve the system both locally and nationally.

The coroner position is a 24/7, 365-days-a-year job. You cannot do this job from behind a desk. You must be willing to be the "boots on the ground" even if it means rolling out of bed at midnight and driving thirty miles over logging roads clogged with snow to investigate an accident scene. You have to do your own "hands-on" investigation from the unique viewpoint of the coroner. Of course, you will get the briefing from the on-scene law enforcement officers. Family members provide valuable information about the deceased, as do other witnesses. My point is that the coroner is the 'ombudsman for the deceased.'

The word autopsy comes from the Greek *autopsis*, "to speak for itself." Kootenai County has about 1300 deaths a year. Approximately 700 of those come under the jurisdiction of the coroner. An autopsy, including toxicology, X-rays, and other tests costs the county approximately $2,500. The present pathology budget is $160,000 a year. Thus, we must select which of those cases we autopsy in order to correctly determine the cause and manner of death. Obviously, we cannot, <u>and should not,</u> autopsy every body which comes to the coroner's office. It requires a delicate balance between the desire to ascertain the cause of death and the financial realities of the budget. The legal responsibility of the coroner "…is to determine the cause and manner of death." Therefore, if the autopsy budget is nearing the annual limit, the coroner must obtain additional funds from the authorizing body, in our case, the Board of County Commissioners (BOCC.) We share this dilemma with just about every coroner/medical examiner office in the United States. My argument to the BOCC is: "…the most expensive autopsy is the one you didn't do and should have done." In addition, the coroner must examine the death certificates before authorizing each cremation. Cremations comprise nearly 70 percent of dispositions in the County.

Law enforcement and the prosecuting attorney make the judgment whether a crime has been committed. They will be responsible for gathering evidence to support their case and deciding whether or not to prosecute. The funeral homes have a pecuniary interest, as well as consoling families. The coroner must determine the cause and manner of death to the exclusion of public perception, family considerations and any efforts to shade the reports to satisfy others.

# CHAPTER 2

# SPOKANE ESTABLISHES A MEDICAL EXAMINER OFFICE

Spokane County and surrounding Eastern Washington counties had a coroner system for many years. Many of the coroners were licensed physicians without formal death investigator training. After a series of well-publicized incidents and miscues, Spokane County hired George Lindholm, MD, a forensic pathologist and established the Spokane County Medical Examiner's Office (SCME) with the actual facility in the Forensic Institute at Holy Family Hospital.

Dr. Lindholm brought a wealth knowledge and experience to the office and fostered good relations with the coroners in North Idaho and Eastern Washington. In addition, he was an established forensic witness who could present expert testimony to the court and juries in clear terms.

Previously, defense attorneys would "attack' the testimony of general pathologists or other physicians as not having sufficient training or expertise in a particular case. This led to the general pathologists being reluctant to do forensic autopsies and have to testify in court. After Dr. Lindholm began his tenure at the Spokane Medical Examiner's Office (SCME), it largely eliminated the difficulty in obtaining forensic autopsies.

Dr. Lindholm's colleagues at the Pathology Associates group readily deferred to his expertise. As a result, most of our forensic autopsies were done at the Spokane facility rather than at Kootenai Medical Center (KMC.) The added transportation costs to and from Spokane were more than offset by the prompt and accurate autopsy results. Dr. Lindholm was most helpful in improving our services in Kootenai County. He occasionally came over to Kootenai County to examine crime scenes or other evidence to enhance his forensic reports.

Subsequently, Sally Aiken, M.D. and John Howard, M.D., continued to elevate the forensic standards of the SCME. Their professional collaboration has greatly assisted the county coroners of North Idaho to provide competent death investigations to determine the cause and manner of death.

As alluded to in a previous chapter, the two SCME forensic pathologists are approaching the caseload limits of their office. The availability of additional forensic medical examiners is limited. Funding concerns will continue to plague both the SCME as well as the Kootenai County Coroner's office. Additionally, obtaining toxicology or DNA results in a timely manner are continuing concerns.

# Chapter 3

# Baptism by Fire

*The body of a beautiful fifteen-year-old ninth grader was discovered in the backyard of a modest home on a Saturday morning in 1973. She had attended a junior high school dance on Friday night, three blocks from her home. Coeur d'Alene police requested the coroner to respond to the scene.*

*She had been strangled and raped. The homeowners had not heard or seen anything unusual during the night. They found the body, and called police.*

*An autopsy disclosed the hyoid bone at the base of the tongue was fractured and other findings were consistent with strangulation. We obtained vaginal samples which showed spermatozoa, nail bed scrapings, clothing and scene photographs.*

*Police investigators interviewed other dance attendees, boyfriends, and other acquaintances. No one noticed other suspicious persons or vehicles in the vicinity of the junior high on the night before the body. One suspect was interviewed at the Montana State Prison, but never charged. He later died in prison.*

The Coeur d'Alene police maintain an open file on this case. The lead detective kept a timeline-white board on his office wall with all of the known details and possible suspects. We would periodically review all of the evidence, without making progress. This was before the advent of DNA samples at autopsy. Whether DNA might have assisted identifying the assailant is unknown. This case haunts the investigating detective and the coroner to this day. It remains a cold case.

*Robert S. West, MD, FACS*

It exemplifies the type of case which occurred in Kootenai County and still perplexes me to this day. This child was subjected to such mindless violence, the police and coroner's office did the investigations, and yet we were unable to track down her assailant.

# Chapter 4

# Planes, Trains, and Automobiles

## Planes

Scheduled airlines use Spokane International Airport as their regional hub. However, private corporate jets and charter flights arrive and depart daily from the Coeur d'Alene Airport (COE). There are 30,000 takeoffs and landings annually with an economic benefit of $150 million dollars. The FAA operates a seasonal air traffic control tower. An instrument landing system and other navigational aids support aircraft operation.

Corporate aircraft from all over the United States and Canada arrive and depart daily. These range from high-performance single and twin-engine aircraft to corporate jet aircraft.

*Air Force-Two,* a Boeing 757, carrying Vice President Cheney, his entourage, and a C-17 with his ancillary support vehicles arrived at COE in a January snowstorm without incident. High profile celebrities, actors, sports figures, and corporate giants regularly show up on the tarmac of this "little" airport.

Empire Airlines does the heavy maintenance for Horizon Airlines, which adds to the mix of aircraft arriving and taking off from COE. The US Forest Service bases firefighting tankers at Coeur d'Alene during the fire season. Tanker bombers load fire retardant and fly missions in a hundred mile radius of Coeur d'Alene. There have been no associated crashes during these busy flying conditions. However, vigilant aircraft maintenance and pilot proficiency is paramount in these operations.

My first exposure to aviation crashes occurred at a private airstrip near Athol, Idaho.

*Several aviation enthusiasts were restoring a WWII vintage DC-3. An evening test flight ended disastrously when the aircraft crashed on takeoff with several casualties. We recovered survivors in trees off the end of the grass runway. The FAA required an autopsy on the pilot to determine if there were underlying medical factors that might have led to the crash. In the end, mechanical failure and pilot error were determined to be the causative factors.*

*Another case involved an instrument-rated, commercial pilot with more than ten thousand hours of flying time. This pilot had flown in the Middle East from Amman, Jordan to Tehran, Iran before the Iran Hostage episode in 1980. After returning to the Pacific Northwest, he was a consultant on cockpit management systems for the Boeing 747 and other commercial aircraft at the Boeing factory in Everett, Washington.*

*He was flying his private twin-engine plane from Everett to Coeur d'Alene for Thanksgiving with two fellow engineers. The weather was marginal, per Instrumental Flight Rules (IFR), with heavy snow and strong westerly winds at forty knots, with gusts to fifty knots.*

*A Cessna Conquest turboprop aircraft landing just prior to him reported low visibility and poor braking conditions due to snow on the runway.*

*The pilot made a non-precision, circling approach to Runway 23. The plane crashed on Hudlow Mountain, about three miles from the approach end of the runway.*

*Sheriff deputies met me on a US Forest Service (USFS) road at the base of the mountain. We clambered up a thirty-degree slope to the still smoldering crash site. After making notes, taking photographs and measurements of the scene, and conferring with the Federal Aviation Administration (FAA) investigator, we removed the victims to funeral vehicles at the base of the mountain.*

*Sometimes, the Coroner is "allowed" to help carry body bags down the mountain. (By the way, I was late for Thanksgiving dinner.)*

*Autopsies showed blunt force trauma with thermal conflagration. The toxicology results showed only elevated levels of carbon monoxide and no illicit substances.*

*Aircraft investigation centered on the aircraft:*

1. Were the engines developing power?
2. Maintenance history and current airworthiness certificate for the aircraft.
3. When was the pilot's most recent flight medical examination and were there any deficiencies?
4. Who was at the controls?

As a private pilot and former senior aviation medical examiner, I ponder the root causes of such accidents: poor decision-making, "get-home-itis," pilot fatigue, and adverse weather, all contributed to this tragic case.

Aviation safety begins with the pre-flight planning, weather briefing, aircraft pre-flight inspection, the actual flight, and does not end until the plane is safely secured after the flight.

Murphy's Law applies to aviation as to other endeavors. Homebuilt, experimental aircraft are especially prone to errors in construction and shortcuts to certification, and frequently exhibit flying characteristics beyond the builder's flying skills.

*One homebuilt aircraft took off from the Coeur d'Alene airport, failed to gain altitude, and crashed in an elementary school playground. Fortunately, school was not in session at the time. The pilot was not as fortunate. FAA investigators determined that a faulty throttle connection was responsible for the crash.*

Powered hang-glider airfoils can fail from metal or fabric fatigue with fatal consequences. Recent creation of the Sport Pilot Category allows pilots with certain medical deficiencies to continue flying, although, they are restricted to non-controlled airspace.

Overall, flying is fundamentally safe. Private airplanes today have more reliable power plants, flight instruments, and navigation equipment than commercial airliners of 1950s vintage. Today's pilot has more training and flight reviews than most drivers on our nation's highways. However, Newton's laws of gravity and inertia are unforgiving and require constant attention if pilots and their passengers are to keep out of the coroner's arena.

*A high-performance single-engine Cessna 210 from Wyoming, carrying six adults, struck trees south of Coeur d'Alene as it descended under IFR on the approach to COE. No one survived, the pilot was decapitated, and the remaining victims sustained multiple mortal injuries. Search and rescue personnel recovered various body parts and the Coroner and Medical Examiner had to match up the body parts before issuing death certificates and releasing the bodies for burial.*

*The weather at the time was overcast with little or no wind or precipitation. Basic pilot error in flight planning, and conduct of the flight led to multiple fatalities.*

*In another instance, a flight service attendant at the Coeur d'Alene airport was struck by a propeller while refueling an airplane. He made it to Kootenai Medical Center, but died in surgery from multiple propeller lacerations.*

Other causes may be more insidious: toxicology from carbon monoxide, alcohol, and various prescription and nonprescription drugs may impair the pilot's ability to control the aircraft.

## Trains

Railroads played a major role in the settlement and development of Idaho. In 1969, railcars filled with lumber still trundled down Front Avenue in downtown Coeur d'Alene. The Spokane Electric Railway brought tourists to a terminus on the waterfront where they boarded steamboats for excursions on the Lake Coeur d'Alene. Ore concentrates from mines in the Silver Valley were loaded at the same site. One derailment near the old Gibbs Lumber Mill on Northwest Boulevard resulted in multiple fatalities.

Most of the rails in Kootenai County are history now, with many of the rail beds converted to bike/pedestrian trails. The Burlington

Northern Santa Fe (BNSF) railroad, however, runs a main line route through Kootenai County. An extensive refueling facility in Rathdrum refuels freight locomotives. Underground fabric barriers and monitoring wells ensure that fuel does not leak into the Rathdrum aquifer.

As many as twenty, one-hundred-car freight trains a day haul coal and crude oil from Montana and North Dakota to Pacific coast terminals. Intermodal freight trains, carrying a variety of cargoes, barrel across the Idaho Panhandle past numerous grade-level railway crossings. Many of these crossings have no barriers and warnings except for the familiar cross-arms. When drivers cross the tracks with their stereo on "high" and the windows rolled up, the result is nearly always tragic.

It takes a mile and a half for a one-hundred-car freight train traveling fifty miles per hour to stop. Locomotive crew-cab videos often show cars driving around lowered cross-arms with lights and bells ringing. It is no wonder these cases result in fatalities.

Alcohol, distracted drivers, and a false sense of security are most often at fault.

*We documented a distraught driver stopped at a crossing for several hours, only to deliberately drive into the path of an oncoming train. That case was classified as suicide after carefully reviewing the history, and examining the victim and vehicle.*

*Another case occurred within the Rathdrum city limits. A van was observed driving erratically, and entered a grade-level crossing where it was struck by a freight train. The driver's autopsy disclosed an acute coronary occlusion. His death was due to the medical incapacitation rather than an accidental death.*

*An intoxicated female sustained a traumatic amputation of her arm and fatal head trauma after she sat on the tracks at another unguarded crossing. We decided to classify her case as an accident on the basis of her blood alcohol level (>.3 gm%.)*

*The "Empire Builder" passenger train makes one eastbound and one westbound pass through North Idaho every day. Although the train makes stops in Sandpoint and Spokane, an unscheduled disembarkation occurs on occasion.*

*Two teenagers on horseback discovered a male body in an advanced state of decomposition along the railroad right-of-way near Post Falls. His trousers were around his ankles but had no other obvious signs of trauma. When identified, the railroad records indicated that he boarded the eastbound Empire Builder in Spokane about six weeks previously. It appeared he was urinating from the platform between cars and fell (or was pushed?) off the train.*

*When the train arrived in Sandpoint, the conductor was notified of the missing passenger. Crews searched the railroad right-of-way from Sandpoint back to Spokane without locating the body. Forensic autopsy, including X-rays did not disclose any external signs of foul play. Larval samples were consistent with the above time frame. The case was classified as accidental even though the possibility exists that the victim might have been pushed from the train.*

The Coroner's Office has worked with Law Enforcement, Idaho Department of Transportation and BNSF to mitigate many of these factors around trains, however, much more needs to be done to reduce the carnage.

## Automobiles

Automobile and truck fatalities are among the most frequent and challenging coroner calls. One of our primary concerns is to *not* become a part of the accident scene. Typically, our response vehicles do not have the flashing lights and identifying markings to distinguish them from other vehicles on scene. My standard practice is to proceed past the accident scene and park ahead of a patrol car or fire truck and well off the shoulder. Far too many secondary accidents and fatalities occur because of inattentive drivers (so-called "Lookee-Sees.")

The majority of our roads are non-divided, two-lane roadways with a high volume of logging trucks, semi-trailers, tractors, other farm machinery, and private vehicles.

Accident scene investigation is the domain of law enforcement. The Coroner's job is to document the position of the victim and the mechanism of injury, and record scene factors that may have contributed to the accident.

Positional asphyxia is best observed before the victim is extricated and may be the only significant injury. Extrication of living injured victims must precede recovery of the deceased body(ies.) This can be a long drawn-out process, but is necessary to ensure the best outcomes.

Much controversy exists over the necessity for forensic autopsies on *all* automobile accident victims. Underlying medical conditions may have contributed to incapacitation prior to the accident. Our on-scene investigation, supplemented by drug and alcohol determinations, helps us make such decisions. Because of the likelihood of litigation or prosecution, most multi-vehicle crash victims are autopsied.

Sudden incapacitation due to a medical condition, such as a heart attack, stroke, seizure, or insulin reaction can be the root cause of an otherwise mysterious crash. One such case involved an anaphylactic reaction to a yellowjacket sting with the driver suddenly losing consciousness and crashing. "Driving while texting" is a relatively recent cause of highway fatalities.

Seat belt use and anti-DUI campaigns have reduced, but not eliminated, the many cases of ejection-type injuries and fatalities. Idaho has one of the highest rates for seatbelt usage in the country.

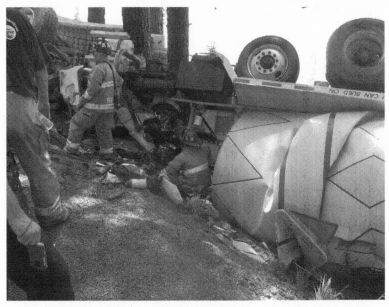

"Cement Truck Rollover, Lake Coeur d'Alene"

*The driver of a fully loaded cement truck lost braking control as he was backing down a steep driveway at a construction site on Lake Coeur d'Alene. The truck overturned with spillage of diesel fuel into the lake. The Idaho Department of Environmental Quality Haz-Mat team supervised the spill control. Medical Personnel extricated the victim from the cab. The driver had received his Commercial Drivers License (CDL) medical exam from the same physician who prescribed his methadone narcotics for back pain. Narcotic use is a specific disqualification for a CDL. Some medical practice behaviors defy common sense and are a threat to public safety.*

*A SWIFT Industries semi-tractor trailer carrying newsprint westbound on I-90 struck the median jersey barrier and overturned. The spilled diesel fuel caught fire. The student commercial truck driver and his instructor sustained massive injuries and were pronounced dead at the scene. The bodies were badly burned. The cause and manner of death were obvious, and toxicology results were negative.*

*The identification papers, truck logs, and other papers were scattered over both lanes of the Interstate for a quarter mile. Idaho State Police recovered one commercial driver's license lying on the pavement.*

*Correct identification required a Forensic Odentologist to match dental records to identify the victims before releasing the bodies to the families for burial. The cause and manner of death were obvious. The toxicology results were negative. It also helped the Idaho State Patrol to determine that the instructor was driving the rig.*

*The National Transportation Safety Board and the Idaho Industrial Commission need to have precise records to process the claims and to assign liability.*

One must not speculate on the circumstances and/or motives of drivers and passengers in all accidents.

*A high-speed rollover on a straight stretch of Highway 41 near Twin Lakes occurred with no other traffic or witnesses. Both out-of-state occupants were ejected from the vehicle and died at the scene. The driver was carrying $2,700 in large denomination bills. Our first suspicions involved a drug deal or some other illegal activity. Upon further investigation, we learned that the men were cleaning apartments for a contractor who paid them in cash just prior to the accident.*

"Suicide by automobile" is an infrequent occurrence, although some circumstances may suggest it as the manner of death. Many drivers entertain suicidal thoughts while driving. Others may act on impulse and drive into a bridge abutment, or over a steep embankment. Unless there is a strong history of depression, other suicidal attempts, or a witness to the event, we tend to err on the side of labeling these cases as accidental.

Domestic arguments may result in one party driving off in a rage and becoming involved in a crash. It is not appropriate to assign suicide as the manner of death in such cases.

The completion of the Veterans Memorial Bridge on I-90 east of Coeur d'Alene has resulted in several victims stopping on the bridge, climbing over the guardrails and jumping to their death on a roadway some 200 feet below. Nearly all of these victims had alcohol or psychiatric issues, or both.

One of the bittersweet aspects of being Coroner in a small community is that eventually, the victim will be someone you know or is somehow related to your life.

*My daughter's high school classmate was killed in a head-on collision on her way home from the University of Idaho. I felt an obligation to go with the Coeur d'Alene police to make notification to the mother.*

*Another fatality involved a physician's son killed in a "wrong way on the freeway" accident involving alcohol (>.34 gm%)*

There are some phone calls you just never want to make.

We investigated several accidents in Hayden Lake involving vehicles driving past well-marked barriers at the Honeysuckle Beach boat launch site.

*One vehicle traveled nearly one hundred yards into the lake before sinking in twenty feet of water. Our problem was to determine who was driving. The victims were not wearing seatbelts. All three of the bodies were in the back seat of the vehicle, probably trying to breathe in an air pocket as the vehicle sank. It is not sufficient to assume that the owner of the vehicle was the driver.*

# Motorcycles, ATVs and Snowmobiles

I have no particular bias for or against any of the above modes of transportation and recreation. Each class of vehicle has some inherent qualities rendering them susceptible to deadly accidents. I do hold the manufacturers and dealers culpable for advertisements which feature extreme driving over rugged terrain and imply that any operator over the age of five should follow suit. There are far too many fatalities to support such notions. Tragically, there are many more cases with traumatic brain injury, quadriplegia or other serious injuries, which never seem to make it into the advertising trailers.

A motorcycle endorsement on your driver's license is required to operate a motorcycle. Idaho only requires helmets for riders seventeen years of age or younger. I fully understand the biker's desire to have "the wind in your hair and the bugs in your teeth."

The laws of physics and gravity apply to motorcycles as much as any other mode of transportation. When a several hundred pound Harley tangles with a 100,000-pound Peterbilt semi-tractor trailer the results are not pretty.

By far, the vast majorities of motorcyclists are very responsible, and share the road with other drivers without incident. Our local weather systems produce inclement driving conditions, which present unique hazards for cyclists.

Living astride the direct route to the annual infamous Sturgis motorcycle gathering, we see an inordinate number of bikers headed to and from South Dakota. To be sure, many of the motorcycles and their gear are worth more than I paid for my home.

*One such group of Oregon bikers rolled into the emergency room of Kootenai Medical Center on a Friday afternoon. A biker had experienced a serious head-on encounter with a car, sustaining serious abdominal trauma and a closed-head injury. We took him to the operating room for emergency surgery. The E.R. and surgical waiting area was flooded with thirty-plus bikers in full leather regalia, fresh (?) from a five-day jaunt with no showers, and raucous in their concern for their fallen "brother."*

*The biker succumbed to his head injury. We ordered a forensic autopsy to ascertain the cause of death, and to document the toxicology results. The "gang" leaders were very insistent that they were going to "return our brother to his motorcycle 'brethren' in Oregon." The Coroner would not release the body until the results were in. Insults were exchanged and gang members implied that no good would come to those standing in their way.*

*Following completion of the autopsy, the body was returned from the Forensic Institute to a local funeral home on Friday evening. The owner of the funeral home, out of town on vacation, was unaware of the conflict.*

*The on-call mortician was at the funeral home on Sunday evening embalming another body for a Monday funeral. He heard the front door slam upstairs and heavy footsteps going from office to office, moving toward the rear stairwell leading to the preparation room. With rising anxiety and a vivid recollection of the gang members' earlier threats, he retrieved his revolver and prepared to "meet the enemy."*

*The unknown "intruder" started down the stairway to the basement area. Heart pounding, the mortician cocked his weapon and prepared to "go down fighting." At that, the owner appeared… narrowly avoiding becoming a statistic, and a coroner case!*

## ATVs

ATV enthusiasts abound on the many trails and roads of North Idaho. Helmet usage is spotty at best, and the further you get into the backwoods, almost non-existent. Fortunately, the geometrically unstable three-wheelers are less common now than they were several years ago. Rollovers and ejection of drivers and/or passengers are often fatal, especially in the un-helmeted cohort. Operator training and safety courses would do much to reduce these accidents and still provide the recreation and sense of the outdoors.

## Snowmobiles

Snowmobilers have access to hundreds of miles of groomed and non-groomed trails stretching across North Idaho to the Montana border. A combination of inadequate winter clothing, the occasional recalcitrant engine, and deep snow may exceed the limits of even the most physically fit operators.

*A group of snowmobilers were engaged in "High Marking" one of the steep bowls in the backcountry. One driver suddenly collapsed. His companions began CPR, which they continued for an hour until medical personnel arrived and pronounced him dead. He suffered a coronary thrombosis, precipitated, in part, by the exertion of snowmobiling.*

## CHAPTER 5

# MISSING PERSONS, UNIDENTIFIED BODIES AND MISSING "PERPS"

### Missing Persons

The National Missing and Unidentified Persons System (NAMUS) is a US Department of Justice (DOJ) national database system for missing persons and/or unidentified bodies. In the past, there was little sharing of missing persons information between agencies or jurisdictions. Now, the Department of Justice will verify such information and post it on the web site. It will contain the person's vital statistics, photo (if available), location, and date last seen. The Web site may have photos, dental information, or significant identification marks. Coroners and medical examiners have access to the system and can add or edit information after suitable training using protected username/passwords.

*On March 29, 1986, Debbie Swanson, a Coeur d'Alene School District #271 Special Education teacher parked her car at the base of Tubbs Hill and went for a hike around the popular trail. She never returned. Her case has been on the NAMUS site for twenty-plus years with no positive hits. The Coeur d'Alene Police Department has kept the case open with available DNA samples to cross match if a possible lead arises.*

The Spokane Medical Examiner now takes DNA samples on every autopsy case to hold on file. At the present time, such samples are not all tested due to financial constraints. In rape and sexual assault cases, however, the samples are tested and entered into an accessible DNA database.

## Unidentified Bodies

We rarely have an unidentified body in Kootenai County. In many of the counties along the southern US border with Mexico, illegal aliens entering the country either succumb to the environment or are victims of assault. At a forensic conference I attended in Scottsdale, Arizona, the Pima County (Tucson) Medical Examiner stated that nearly one hundred bodies each year remain unidentified after autopsy, DNA, fingerprinting and dental X-Rays.

In 2004, the Department of Justice, Bureau of Justice Statistics reported that there were 4,400 unidentified bodies in two thousand U.S. Coroner offices. One thousand were still unidentified after one year.

Any unidentified bodies are entered in the NAMUS database using the above parameters. The availability of the database information in many cases has established the identity of the victim and provided closure for families.

## Unclaimed Persons

A recent additional NAMUS category is the Unclaimed Persons section. These are bodies whose names and identities are known, but have no known next of kin or responsible person to claim the body for disposition. I am not certain whether the current economic climate or other social changes are responsible for this rising new category. I do know that in 2009, the Wayne County (Detroit) Medical Examiner's office had a crisis in "unclaimed bodies" with dozens of unclaimed bodies in the Wayne County morgue and with nobody to claim them for disposition.

Two examples of the NAMUS database's use involve a double homicide in Athol, Idaho, and a shooting victim on a bridge near Coeur d'Alene.

In the first case, a mother and daughter were shot to death by the husband/father. He was last seen driving northbound on U.S. Highway 95, but it was never determined whether he drove into one of the panhandle lakes or entered Canada. We broadcast his vehicle, license number and physical description to Canadian officials and U.S. Border Patrol and Customs. We entered his Vital Statistics in NAMUS and the National Crime Information Center (NCIC) system.

Records showed that the family did upholstery repairs in their home, the sixteen-year-old daughter worked part-time at the Silverwood Amusement Park. KCSO reported prior domestic disturbance calls from the residence.

A .22-caliber rifle was recovered at the scene. The ballistics matched the slugs recovered from both victims. The case remains open. The NCIC file has not had any hits in several years. There was an unconfirmed report of a person possibly matching his description appearing at the Canadian/US border crossing at Porthill. It was not confirmed however.

The second case involved a male body dumped on the Blue Creek Bridge, east of Coeur d'Alene in the westbound lanes of I-90. The victim was nearly headless from a gunshot wound to the face. Fortunately, police were able to trace the killing to the Portland, Oregon, area through an all-points bulletin issued by the Portland Metropolitan Police. We never could determine why the victim was dumped in the westbound lanes, or why they did not dump the body over the bridge into Lake Coeur d'Alene.

Positive identification through fingerprints, blood typing and DNA provided the necessary match for Portland law enforcement. This case is another example of cooperation of multiple agencies to apprehend criminals even in Coeur d'Alene, Idaho.

# CHAPTER 6

# MARINE ISSUES

The Idaho Panhandle is blessed with a multitude of lakes, rivers, and streams. Over 45,000 acres of the surface area of Kootenai County are water. The St. Joe River flowing into the southern end of Lake Coeur d'Alene is the highest-elevation commercially navigable river in the world. During the timber industry's heyday, tugboats towing huge rafts of logs in excess of five million board-feet of lumber would take thirty-six to forty-eight hours to come up the lake to log-storage areas near several large lumber mills in Coeur d'Alene.

Boaters returning from the "watering holes" in Carlin Bay and Rockford Bay would encounter the lighted booms of logs, or strike the towline stretching for hundreds of yards behind the tugboat. The occupants would either end up high and dry on the log booms, or drown as the boat sank. Most of these victims were never recovered from the lake.

Cruise boats have plied the waters of Lake Coeur d'Alene for more than a hundred years. They offer a delightful way to see the sights, cruise up the "shadowy St. Joe River" and offer genuine relaxation. They also host many party excursions and libations in liberal amounts. College students from the University of Idaho at Moscow, Idaho, and Washington State University in Pullman, Washington, come by the hundreds with typical recreational aspirations. Bartenders on the boats will "shut off" obviously intoxicated passengers for their own safety. "Binge drinking" happens on the water as well as on campus.

Occasionally, a drunken, belligerent passenger will threaten to jump overboard if not served.

There are *no* categories of "terminal stupidity" or "dead drunk" to list as the cause of death. For years, we classified these cases as suicides. I have gradually modified my thinking after consulting with various forensic pathologists and law enforcement. I now classify most of these as accidental deaths. Preventable to be sure, but often with a blood alcohol level in excess of 0.45 gm%, the victim is *not capable* of deciding to commit suicide. I realize not all medical examiners/coroners will agree with me, however, that has worked in Kootenai County.

*    *    *

The depth of Lake Coeur d'Alene exceeds 200 feet in places. There is a gradual south-to-north current to the outlet at the Spokane River near North Idaho College. Bodies that sink below the thermocline level do not surface from the processes of putrefaction. The Marine Department of the Kootenai County Sheriff's office uses side-scanning sonar to identify objects on the lake bottom, including sunken steamers, Model T Fords, bicycles, and the occasional body. Numerous sunken logs and other debris make determining the search location crucial.

*When an individual jumped from a motorboat coming up the lake at night, several 911 cell phone calls came in alerting the marine division. A sailboat in the area tried to recover the victim, to no avail. Eyewitnesses gave a location just off Arrow Point at one of the narrowest and deepest portions of the lake. The Marine Division made a methodical grid search with the sonar equipment without any likely target. Using GPS triangulation, the 911 center traced the cell phone calls to various cell towers in the area and established a position more than a half-mile north of the eyewitness's location. When the sonar scan moved to the more northerly location, the body was soon located in 130 feet of water. Scuba divers were unable to retrieve the victim at that depth.*

*A civic-minded couple from Kuna, Idaho, with a remote operating vehicle (ROV), responded. They provide lake retrieval services throughout Idaho on a volunteer basis, asking for only mileage and fuel reimbursement.*

*The ROV was able to descend along the buoy marker line with real-time video surveillance to the body. Its "grasper" arm clamped down on the victim's arm. The body and the ROV were winched to the surface. Rescue swimmers secured a line to the body which was then secured to the transom of the KCSO marine vessel and transported to the KCSO boathouse. We made identification by tattoos and clothing to confirm the identity of the drowning victim.*

Recovery of drowning victims provides closure for families and is a part of the function of the Coroner's Office. We salute the Kuna volunteers for their assistance in these cases.

*In another instance, a couple was operating their large cruiser at night near Carlin Bay. According to the wife, her husband was standing on the swim platform working on the drive unit. He fell into the lake and drowned. The circumstances were unusual in that the wife stated she was mixing her husband a cocktail, and when she brought the drink to the cockpit, her husband was gone. The wife was unfamiliar with the operation of the large boat.*

*Her delay in notifying authorities, though, made the exact location difficult to determine. Eventually, the KCSO and the Kuna ROV unit located and retrieved the body.*

*An autopsy did not reveal any traumatic injuries and a moderately elevated blood alcohol level. We listed the cause of death as accidental fresh-water drowning.*

In 2011, the KCSO Marine Division acquired an ROV, and has begun acquiring the skills and procedures for its operation.

The visual clarity of the video and the maneuverability of the grasper arm are truly remarkable. It is one of those technological marvels never imagined in years past. It is one thing to see an ROV hovering over the *RMS Titanic* or the Deepwater Horizon Oil Well spill in the Gulf of Mexico. It is entirely another to see this technology in use in Kootenai County.

*Lake Coeur d'Alene rarely freezes over in winter. When it does, an entirely new set of hazards comes into play. "Old-timers" speak of the lake freezing over and people driving their Model-T Fords down to the town of Harrison some twenty miles south. The number of Model T relics on the lake bottom bear witness to such stories.*

*In 1975, the last time the lake froze over, I ruefully admit to joining such foolhardy behavior. When the lake is frozen, residents in the boat-access only portion of Casco Bay are isolated. Fred Murphy, a venerable tugboat operator, would punch a channel in the ice from his lake home to town with his tugboat. When the ice thickness made that impossible, the ever-resourceful Fred and his son ran snowmobiles across the ice, building an "ice road" as snow piled on the ice. After several inches of snow had fallen, the trail became well packed down. Then, it rained and the weather turned very cold.*

*This intrepid Coroner, his wife, our daughter and her fiancé decided to cross-country ski the "ice road" to our cabin in Casco Bay. About two-thirds of the way to Murphy's home, we tracked off the 'ice road' to cut across to the cabin. We immediately encountered wet snow over a couple of inches of water on top of the underlying ice layer. Our skis caked up with snow and ice. Fortunately, none of us broke through the ice, probably thanks to the distribution of our weight on the skis. We were soaking wet by the time we got to the cabin. We started a fire, but it became clear that our clothes would not dry out before darkness set in.*

*In our damp clothes, we set out and tracked along the shore until we reached the 'ice road' at the Murphy home, where we started back across the lake to Coeur d'Alene. We finally reached the city—cold, hypothermic, and thoroughly chastened. We were thankful to be alive. I admit poor judgment on my part, inexcusable for a North Dakota native. ["Confession is the better part of valor!"]*

Tragically, Fred Murphy became another victim of Lake Coeur d'Alene when he drowned after his snowmobile crashed through the ice.

Pend Oreille Lake is another matter. The southern end of Lake Pend Oreille reaches depths of 1,250 feet. Thousands of years ago, glaciers scoured the lakebed down to the basalt. Recurring glacial plugs dammed the Clark Fork River impounding Glacial Lake Missoula to a depth of 2,000 feet behind the dam, and containing an estimated 500 cubic *miles* of water.

About 10,000 years ago, the last of several "Glacial Outburst Floods" occurred. Geologists term these events "Jokulhlaups," an Icelandic term adapted into English language. The huge Glacial Lake Missoula drained in a matter of several days resulting in a massive 1,000-foot wall of water traveling at sixty to one hundred miles per hour surging out over the Rathdrum Prairie, past Spokane leaving huge "erratic" boulders on the scablands of Eastern Washington. It finally spilled down the Columbia River and emptied into the Pacific Ocean.

Boats offshore on current Lake Pend Oreille may be in 900+ feet of water. Thousands of former sailors from the nearby Farragut Naval Training Center will attest that the water temperature is never more than 50 degrees. Water from Lake Pend Oreille percolates through the gravels of the Rathdrum Aquifer, which supplies pure drinking water to hundreds of thousands of people in the Inland Northwest. Deep wells tap irrigation water for agricultural purposes as well. Eventually, the aquifer empties into the Spokane River.

The KCSO sonar equipment is unable to search below 700 feet due to winch cable capacity. Drowning victims have been followed down to 700 feet only to lose the image. The United States Navy Research facility at Bayview, Idaho, tests submarine sonar and propulsion systems in the lake far from the searching eyes of real or potential enemies. Their sonar and ROVs may have greater capabilities, but that data is classified and not available to civilian agencies.

Boats in distress on Pend Oreille cannot look to the Naval Research facility for assistance.

*In one instance, a propane heater on a fishing boat caught fire, which quickly engulfed the boat in flames. One of the occupants, wearing a life jacket, was rescued by a nearby boat. A second swimmer managed to make it to the naval barge where he was promptly detained by naval security forces. The other occupant drowned and the body was never recovered. Because it was a witnessed drowning, we issued a death certificate with the cause of death listed as "freshwater drowning; manner, accidental."*

*In another case, a couple from Spokane spent the night on their cabin cruiser moored at the Bayview marina. The next morning, the wife was missing from the boat. All of her belongings remained on the boat. The couple's car was still in the parking lot. All evidence pointed to a presumed drowning. KCSO investigators handled the case, took photographs of the boat and dock area, and interviewed the husband and marina personnel.*

*We deferred issuing a death certificate because of the circumstances and lack of witnesses to the actual drowning. The usual procedure is to present the evidence to a judge who can sign an order directing the Coroner to issue a death certificate. That case is under judicial review at the time of this writing.*

In some cases, either the manner or the cause of death may be listed as "Cannot be determined." In the event that evidence is discovered for a definite cause or manner of death, the death certificate can be amended once but only once. [I will discuss death certificates in a later chapter.]

While this may cause problems for the family and others involved in the matter of the estate, experience has led me to be very careful about certifying a death without a body or actual witnesses exist.

*Case in point: Two hunters were out duck hunting on one of the bays on Lake Coeur d'Alene. They had decoys, shotguns, and a Labrador retriever in a flat bottomed "duck boat." We found the boat adrift with all of their equipment, guns and the dog. Their vehicle was still parked at the launching area, but no sign of either hunter.*

*To make matters worse, his wife was an operating room (OR) nurse at Kootenai Medical Center. We consoled and grieved with her as the investigation continued for several months.*

*She alluded to some financial difficulties, but nothing major. There was a subtle sense that we had not gotten the entire story. Investigators continued their searches. We entered the hunter's physical descriptions and vital statistics into the National Missing and Unidentified Persons System (NAMUS) database. The "widow" continued her duties at the hospital. To casual observers, she seemed to be "holding up" well.*

*Three months later, both missing hunters were located in Colorado and their elaborate hoax unraveled. They returned to face charges in Kootenai County. The nurse left Kootenai Medical Center shortly thereafter.*

\*    \*    \*

*In the late 1970s, two teenagers visiting a noncustodial relative were lounging on air mattresses in Bennett's Bay on Lake Coeur d'Alene. A powerboat, towing a water skier, drove over them. The boy drowned. We were not able to recover his body.*

*I was the on-call surgeon when the young female was brought into the emergency room at Kootenai Medical Center. Only a small tag of skin attached her lower leg to the upper thigh, which also had several deep propeller lacerations. I consulted with an Orthopedic Surgeon, and we determined the lower leg was not salvageable. She was resuscitated with fluids and blood transfusions. She was started on antibiotics and a tetanus booster administered. Because neither parent was available to give consent, we used an emergency witnessed consent, signed by both consultants. We performed a below-knee amputation and repaired her other lacerations.*

This patient returned to my office several years later fully ambulatory with her B/K prosthesis, and thankful for the care she received at Kootenai Medical Center.

\*     \*     \*

Scuba diving accidents present another challenge for the Coroner. Scuba instructors from Coeur d'Alene and Spokane bring classes to the lake for an "Open Water" dive experience. They participate in periodic lake-bottom clean-up activities, and dive to several sunken steamboats around the lake.

*An open-water dive in January ended tragically. Jim West [no relation], a master certified diver from Spokane, was conducting a "dry suit" dive when his student diver suddenly surfaced from about a 60-foot depth. The compensator valve on her suit malfunctioned and sent her to the surface, resulting in bronchial rupture and air embolism.*

*The information we gave to the SCME Forensic Lab gave them a heads-up for special techniques to use to confirm our suspicions of air in the right atrium of the heart.*

*Another contract diver employed by the Coeur d'Alene Resort Golf Course was retrieving some of the hundreds of golf balls on the lake bottom beneath the fourteenth hole floating green. Although certified, he had not dived for more than a year, was obese and in poor physical condition.*

*A malfunction in his scuba gear failed to deliver oxygen to him. He was unable to surface in time to prevent drowning. We also considered a possible problem with the air tank. He had filled his air tanks at a Coeur d'Alene Fire Station using an air compressor without a water vapor barrier.*

This industrial accident triggered an OSHA and Idaho Industrial Commission investigation. The tanks tested negative for carbon monoxide. Occasionally, exhaust from a gasoline powered air compressor containing carbon monoxide may get into the air intake mixing with the compressed air in the tank and causing the diver to succumb to carbon monoxide poisoning. Testing for carbon monoxide in the above case was negative.

A motto we strive to follow is "Know what you know. More importantly, know what you do not know!"

When investigating a case with law enforcement the last question should always be, "What else?" You need to ask, "Have I done all of the investigation possible? Is there some piece of evidence we have overlooked that might have some bearing on the case?"

For several years, I shared office space with an Internist/Hematologist named Marvin Powell, M.D. Fellowship trained and famously social he was a valued colleague and friend. We enjoyed many years of differing, practices. He shared with me the story of an industrialist who decided to retire from the pressures of his Connecticut-based Tool and Die business.

*The "Connecticut Yankee" was building a mountaintop retreat near Rose Lake, Idaho, on a lot sold to him by Jim Ratliff, a Coeur d'Alene Realtor. Ratliff sold both Marv and I our homes in Coeur d'Alene. Our families were close friends. The Connecticut Yankee seemed to have abundant cash resources for the land and building project. He had dinner with Marv and Jim at their homes. Dr. Powell was seeing him for a lymphoma previously treated by radiation in Connecticut.*

*In short, he resembled numerous other refugees from the "urban rat-race." The Realtor and Dr. Powell entertained the man on his periodic trips from Connecticut to North Idaho. This went on for several months.*

*One winter evening, Jim Ratliff received a phone call from a person identifying himself as an FBI agent. The agent wanted to know whether*

*Ratliff knew this individual. Wary of strangers calling for such information, Ratliff initially declined to give out any specifics. The agent said, "I'm going to hang up now. You get the FBI number from the Coeur d'Alene phone book and call me back."*

*As it turned out, our "industrialist" had indeed been building a retreat in the mountains near Rose Lake, Idaho. He was using the proceeds from numerous bank heists in New York and Connecticut to fund his real estate and building venture. Furthermore, on his return trips to New York, he was carrying dynamite procured from an explosives plant in Hayden, Idaho.*

Remember, this was well before Oklahoma City or 9/11. This was money laundering before money laundering was invented.

*He was captured in Connecticut during one bank robbery. During his trial, he managed to overpower and shoot a court bailiff plus several others in the courtroom. He made his escape in a hail of gunfire. The FBI had information that he was trying to make it to his mountain retreat in Idaho.*

*A posse consisting of Sheriff's Deputies, FBI, and assorted other agencies headed up the mountains on snowmobiles to the cabin. Guns drawn, they approached the cabin that commanded a 360-degree view of the terrain. The cabin was vacant. However, the FBI and KCSO found a well-fortified retreat with enough ammunition and food to hold off an army for several months. The robber was later captured in Connecticut.*

Lessons learned:

1. Do not believe everything you are told.
2. Trust and verify.
3. Realtors may not have all the information on their clients.

# CHAPTER 7

# INDIGENOUS AND EXOTIC SPECIES HAZARDS

One of North Idaho's many attractions is the absence of poisonous snakes. I grew up in rattlesnake country in North Dakota. When I was four years old, my dad killed a rattlesnake on the front porch of our farmhouse where I had been making "mud pies." We learned never to put your foot down without first looking for a snake. My dad also made an emergency exit from our outhouse with his bib-overalls at half-mast when a rattler buzzed just as he sat down!

I fully appreciate the value of snakes in the control of vermin like rats and mice. The prairie dog town near our farm was probably an attractive food source for them. Nevertheless, I have a certain visceral reaction to reptiles that I will never lose.

*An internist in the office building where I practiced had a pet boa constrictor. He became quite depressed over multiple domestic problems, and had several odd mannerisms. One day, he brought a chest x-ray to my office. He pointed to the cardiac shadow and said that he thought that would be the correct place to place a bullet. Regrettably, I failed to recognize the X-ray as his, and the implications of his intentions.*

*Less than a week later, I responded to his residence for a suicide call. When I arrived at the home on Blackwell Hill, my first question to the investigating police officer was: "Where is the snake?" I could handle the details of investigating the suicide, but I did not want to have a five-foot boa constrictor mosey out from behind a couch while we were in the house. We later determined the doctor had disposed of the snake.*

In 2010, a reclusive man in Rathdrum, Idaho, called the police asking for medical assistance. A convicted felon, he had moved there after his release from prison. Aside from some "crank" calls about his radical ideas about society and people trespassing on his property, the police had had little contact with him. He had severe Chronic Obstructive Pulmonary Disease (COPD) and was under the care of the Veterans Administration (VA) Hospital in Spokane.

He stated he would meet the officer and paramedics on his front porch and, furthermore, they were not to enter his house. The ambulance arrived and promptly transported him to Kootenai Medical Center where, unfortunately, he died. His estranged family lived in Pittsburgh, Pennsylvania. They were not interested in coming to claim his personal effects. They directed the police to ship his household items to Pennsylvania. When Officers gained entry to the house, they found a menagerie of exotic animals including several pythons, an iguana, several large scorpions plus a supporting cast of rats, mice and rabbits representing the "menu."

The Rathdrum police officer had an aversion to snakes akin to mine. He contacted Panhandle Pet Rescue, an organization primarily involved with stray cats and dogs. The woman who responded was acquainted with the man and his exotic pet collection. She proceeded to capture and take several of the snakes, iguana, and scorpions, as well as the "menu" animals to their facility. As she left, she told officers: "I couldn't find the nine-foot python I gave him about three months ago." They searched the house again without finding the snake.

When I returned from a forensic medicine seminar in Scottsdale, Arizona, Jody DeLuca Hissong, my Chief Deputy Coroner, related the story to me. I called the Rathdrum police and talked to the officer who had first responded to the call. He was not interested in making another trip to that house. He said, "Doc, I really do not like snakes!" I responded: "What if there is a python in the house and some stranger or kid gets in there when the python is really hungry? Do me a favor, have the Panhandle Pet Rescue lady go through the house with you one more time."

*He reluctantly agreed to do so. About two hours later, I got the call: "Okay, Doc, there was a nine foot long Burmese python behind a desk in the living room."*

*Panhandle Rescue removed the reptile and both of us slept better that night.*

As the reader may be aware, pythons and other exotic species have escaped or been released into the Everglades National Park in Florida. They have established a breeding population of pythons estimated at more than 100,000 in Florida alone. Pythons have no natural predators and the result has been the decimation of numerous indigenous species including deer, alligators, wild boar, and numerous small mammals. This threatens the entire ecosystem of the Everglades. Specimens up to nineteen feet have been captured during State Fish And Wildlife Department-authorized hunts.

I have no idea whether pythons would survive in the climatic conditions in the Idaho Panhandle. I personally am not interested in finding out!

*WRB was another recluse living near Athol, Idaho. He once berated a postal carrier who came to check on his welfare after he had not picked up his mail for several days. Neighbors respected his right to privacy. When several weeks went by in February 2008, KCSO was notified and made a welfare check.*

*They discovered WRB deceased on the floor of the home. The wood stove, used for heat, was cold. A domestic cat, left without food or water had consumed a substantial portion of his head and neck. There were no other signs of foul play, and the house was otherwise undisturbed. Relatives from out-of-state were located and claimed his remains.*

# CHAPTER 8

# HUNTERS AND THE HUNTED

Big game and big game hunters abound in Northern Idaho. The forests of Kootenai County have all the major species: deer, elk, wolves, coyotes, moose, black bear, grizzly bear, cougar, and bobcats. The grizzly bear and woodland caribou are federally protected species, as are a small population of wolverine and lynx. The Scotsman Peaks in the Cabinet Mountain wilderness area in Bonner County also have a protected mountain goat population. It is pure speculation whether hunters outnumber game during hunting season. Gun safety and hunter education programs are crucial to the sport. However, we still investigate a number of hunting accidents every year.

*A year after I came to Coeur d'Alene, several Kootenai Medical Center staff members were hunting in the Lolo National Forest near St. Regis, Montana. Another non-resident hunter fired a "sound shot" (firing through brush toward the sounds of movement) and struck an orthopedic surgeon in the chest. The doctor died before he could be transported to a medical facility.*

The range and muzzle velocity of present-day weapons make it imperative to "know your target and everything beyond it."

Carrying loaded weapons in vehicles is an invitation for disaster. Many accidents occur in the process of exiting or entering vehicles. Likewise, the process of unloading weapons prior to placing them into the vehicle may result in an unintended discharge. The Coroner and law enforcement must decide whether a given case represents an accident, manslaughter (homicide), or even suicide. Law enforcement and the County Prosecutor make the determination whether or not a case warrants manslaughter charges.

When you add in the effects of alcohol, other drugs, and the physical and medical condition of the victim, and the process becomes even more complex.

Additionally, in the majority of cases the victim has been moved or the crime/accident scene disturbed. The accident site may be dozens of miles from Coeur d'Alene and only accessible by foot or horseback. Improvisation becomes the order of the day. Preserving the evidence, securing the firearm, and extensive use of photographs of the scene, even recording the GPS coordinates allows investigators to reconstruct the incident. Whenever possible, each victim should be tagged, protective bags placed over the hands, and the transport pouch secured before transport. The forensic lab can then determine whether to do ballistic residue testing under controlled conditions. Personal effects can be examined and catalogued at the lab, as well as a search for other substances which might have some bearing on the case.

Hunter vs. hunted role-reversal has been a rare occurrence. Cougars, although secretive, have stalked hunters without any recent attacks in Idaho. There are instances of hikers and joggers being attacked by cougars in areas surprisingly close to urban locations in Colorado, Washington state and elsewhere.

Martha and I encountered a mother black bear and two cubs on a hike up behind our Casco Bay cabin. We were downwind from her and a light rain was falling. We stood stock-still for about fifteen minutes while momma and her cubs sauntered up the hillside out of sight. I am confident that we would never have been able to outrun her if she had charged. Martha was *not* amused by my comment that I only needed to outrun *her*! She has never again suggested a hike in that area.

Migratory waterfowl hunting, on the many lakes and rivers in Kootenai County, has its own hazards. Fall weather can be unpredictable with wet, rainy and cold conditions; high wind-chill factors, blustery winds, and shorter periods of daylight. Snowstorms and weather systems can develop rapidly, despite no weather predictions of inclement conditions.

Foul-weather gear, waders and decoys loaded in a marginally stable flat-bottomed boat or kayak leave a scant margin of safety for hunters. Hypothermia and cold-water shock can result in drowning in less than four feet of water. Surprisingly, when a boat flips (usually occasioned by the recoil of a shotgun resulting in sudden movement and capsizing the boat) hunters often attempt to swim to shore in water that may be only waist deep. Cold-water survival instructors use the "50-50-50 Rule." You have a 50 percent chance of surviving 50 minutes in 50-degree water. That is, if you are stone cold sober, and in top physical condition.

The camouflage and concealment used by wild turkey hunters has its own hazard when trigger-happy hunters fail to identify their target.

Upland game hunting is largely confined to the Palouse Country and Hells Canyon population of chukar, pheasant, and grouse. The steep terrain in the prime chukar areas is physically challenging for even well-conditioned hunters. Sedentary, couch-potato nimrods who attempt to follow a retriever on the scent of a covey of chukars are candidates for the heart-stopping "Big One."

Moose hunting is permitted with lottery-drawn, non-transferable tags. Hunters can have only one tag in a lifetime.

*We encountered an individual brought to Kootenai Medical Center in critical condition after an auto collision. He sustained multiple chest and abdominal injuries in addition to extremity fractures. Emergency Room personnel began immediate fluid resuscitation with IV fluids, blood transfusions. Bilateral chest tube insertion produced frank blood in large quantities. A distended abdomen and free air under the diaphragm indicated a ruptured hollow viscus. The unconscious patient's vital signs continued to deteriorate despite massive transfusions of uncrossmatched blood. His condition never stabilized sufficiently to take him to the operating room. Cardiac arrest ensued and resuscitation efforts proved futile. The patient expired.*

*Family members including his wife had arrived at the hospital. Nurses kept them in a private waiting area and kept them apprised of the patient's* status. As the attending surgeon, I made the dreaded walk to the waiting area to break the news to the new widow and her family.

There were many tears and much grief as I described our futile efforts to stabilize him and that, unfortunately, he was now deceased.

The wife naturally shocked and grief stricken, suddenly stopped crying, looked up at me, and said: "Well, just **WHO** is going to fill his moose tag?"

The E.R. nurse and I tried, unsuccessfully, to maintain our "game faces." We backed out of the room until we could recover our composure.

Eventually, we were able to console her and the family, realizing the inappropriate response was a result of emotional shock.

# CHAPTER 9

# NOTHING LIKE A WALK IN THE WOODS

This brings me to one of the most fascinating coroner cases I have ever experienced in Kootenai County. It illustrates the close cooperation between multiple agencies and the dogged pursuit of a heinous criminal through the meticulous acquisition of evidence to successfully prosecute the perpetrator. It also highlights the forensic complexities a coroner faces when you must have the ability to facilitate a complex investigation utilizing resources that go well beyond those available in the local community.

Hunting in the fall is a magical time. The leaves are off the aspens, the crisp fall air is mixed with the aroma of pines. You expect frequent deer, moose, and occasional elk sightings.

*On Friday, October 6, 2000, two young quail hunters shuffled up a draw less than a quarter mile from a makeshift campsite on the USFS road. One of them kicked over some leaves and a jawbone. At first, thinking it was from a deer, they picked it up. There were dental fillings! No deer sports dental fillings. This was definitely human.*

*They brought it to the Kootenai County Sheriff's Office at about 4:30 p.m. My very good friend and colleague, Detective Brad Maskell took one look at the specimen and said, "Houston, we have a problem!"*

*Detective Maskell went back to the original undeveloped campsite with the hunters to localize the site and determine a search area. He set up a command post at the campsite and established 24-hour security. Crime scene tape barred access to the area. During the rest of the weekend, Kootenai Search and Rescue assembled a team of searchers and briefed them on a search protocol. They combed the draw for a mile upstream, and the hillsides on either side in a grid search pattern. The terrain is steep and heavily wooded, with numerous deadfalls in the uneven ground. The process was slow and tedious.*

*Shortly, however, they began to find more skeletal remains scattered over a large area on the hilltop to the east of the draw. Each bone was photographed in situ ( in place,) a numbered marker placed, and the individual bones placed in paper sacks and sealed. They located a femur, an intact pelvis, ribs, ulnae, a radius, and several cervical and thoracic vertebrae. They found the skull, minus the previous mentioned jawbone, near a fallen tree. Nearby, a blood-stained commemorative tee shirt from the 1995-96 deployment of the USS Nimitz, an aircraft carrier based in Everett, WA They also recovered a large piece of mummified, leathery skin with several incised wounds, and evidence of animal chewing around the edges. Many of the bones also showed evidence of carnivores chewing on the fragments.*

*Eventually, they recovered nearly 80% of the skeleton from an area the size of three football fields draped over the brow of the hill and down either side. Detective Maskell and two deputies brought the skull to my office the following Monday. They described the events above.*

*Upon examining the skull and jawbone, it matched completely. I noticed several larval forms coming out of the suture lines on the top of the skull. These tiny bugs, known as "cheese skippers," were not at all like the larval (maggots) forms seen in typical decomposing bodies. We recovered several of the larvae plus several empty egg cases (pupae) from the interior of the skull and placed them in 70% alcohol preservative solution. We placed all of the recovered skeletal remains in cold storage to defer further maturation of the larvae.*

*Detective Maskell, the Spokane Medical Examiner, and I began the process of identification. Missing person reports for Kootenai and Spokane County were reviewed. A NAMUS search turned up no hits. Dr. Neil Boaz, Ph.D., a Forensic Anthropologist at Eastern Washington University,*

*Cheney, WA., Kathy Taylor, Ph.D., the Washington State Forensic Anthropologist; and Dr. Frank Morgan, DDS, a Forensic Odentologist, examined the skull and jawbone. The pelvis was clearly female with a non-fused pubic symphysis; the jawbone and skull had four unerupted third molars, in addition to the restorations noted above. Several non-fused epiphyses on the long bones indicated a female, 14-16 years old. We noted several incised marks on two of the cervical vertebrae. Numerous rodent marks were present on nearly all of the bones.*

*Attempts at rehydration of the mummified skin fragment for DNA or fingerprints were not successful. It appeared to be from the lower back area.*

*I contacted Neal Haskell, PhD, a renowned Forensic Entomologist at Rensslaer University in Indiana, for suggestions on further studies. He suggested I try to obtain additional pupae cases, or other larval stages, from the scene. I accompanied a KCSO deputy approximately 26 miles into the National Forest to the command post/campsite. The security deputy there allowed us into the area. We clambered up the steep hillside to the numbered markers where the skeletal remains were recovered. I recovered several pupae cases and other debris, and placed them in plastic bags, labeled and sealed them.*

*We then shipped these bags, along with the skull larvae, to Dr. Haskell for analysis. In addition, I was able to get climate data from the USFS Weather Station at Fernan for the six months preceding, showing daily high/low temperatures, humidity, and weather observations in the Coeur d'Alene area.*

*Dr. Haskell's report estimated that death had occurred at least five months previously, based on the larval species recovered and the climatic data for the period. The progression of species found in decomposing bodies follows a typical pattern. These patterns have been extensively documented at the "Body Farm" at Vanderbilt University in Nashville, Tennessee. Dr. Haskell has confirmed those studies in his own research and practice.*

*Detectives discovered a missing person/runaway report of a fourteen-year-old girl in Post Falls, Idaho. Last seen on July 2, 2000, she had been reported missing by her mother. Her dental x-rays and dental records were compared to our skull and jawbone, and they matched. The skeleton now had a name: Carissa Benway.*

*The following paraphrased excerpts come from a narrative prepared by Detective Maskell, and were compiled from multiple interviews with David "Coon" Merritt, his son Cody, and other known acquaintances of the missing girl.*

*Carissa was a student at Post Falls Middle School. She was a "fair" student, who had several minor juvenile offenses. She and several other friends began frequenting the mobile home belonging to David "Coon" Merritt in the Chateau Trailer Park in Post Falls, Idaho. Coon and his son, Cody, watched TV with the teenagers, and furnished them with alcohol, marijuana, and other drugs. He referred to them as his "puppies."*

*"Coon" worked as a chef at a restaurant in Coeur d'Alene. He was a convicted sex offender out on parole. He boasted that he was a member of a motorcycle gang known as 'The Brotherhood' and he had considered himself a "bad-ass." He sported a Black Rose Tattoo on his right arm with a scroll inscribed with "Brotherhood" beneath it. He stated that tattoo was reserved for gang members who either had killed someone, or watched someone be killed.*

*He became attracted to Carissa and jealous whenever Cody and Carissa would hug and kiss on a couch in the living room of the trailer.*

*"Coon" photographed the teens in various poses including simulated or actual sexual situations. He encouraged them to flash their breasts for photos. He began asking Carissa to pose for photographs in his USS Nimitz tee shirt and a patterned sweater later found at the crime scene. He once told Cody to destroy the pornographic pictures, as they broke the conditions of his parole.*

*Carissa Benway accompanied "Coon" and Cody Merritt on a camping trip over the Fourth of July weekend in 2000. She brought her earnings from selling magazine subscriptions for a company in the Spokane Valley. Coon paid for her $80 taxi fare from Spokane to Post Falls. They picked up a tent, sleeping bags, and a .22-caliber rifle at a friend's house. They stopped for groceries and other supplies at the Silver Lake Mall, and headed up into the Panhandle National Forest in a crew-cab pickup. Carissa, wearing only a swimsuit bra and bottoms, slept in the back seat of the pickup on the way to a secluded campsite about a mile from the developed USFS Honeysuckle*

Campground. The developed campgrounds in the National Forests are heavily utilized in the summer months, especially on the July 4 weekend.

The trio selected an undeveloped campsite. They set up their tent, got a fire going, and cooked dinner. Cody and Carissa went for a short hike up the draw. Cody noted that Coon maintained a close watch on them as if to prevent them from running away.

Cody tended the campfire. He was told to stand guard in case a car stopped at the campsite. At gunpoint, Coon took Carissa into the tent, secured her wrists to a pole with Zip Ties, and proceeded to rape and sodomize her for more than two hours. Later, Cody went into the tent. The trio slept, with Carissa as far from Coon as possible. Carissa had only a small blanket to wrap around herself because Coon had cut off her bra and swimsuit bottoms during the attack.

The next morning, Cody saw Coon secreting a large knife sheathed in cardboard in the back of his jeans. Coon said, "It's time." They took Carissa up the draw and climbed partway up the hillside. As Cody looked back, he saw Coon grab Carissa by the hair, hyper-extend her neck, and slash her throat from right to left. Her carotid arteries and jugular veins spurted blood. Terrified, when she attempted to breathe, the only sound was the gurgle of air escaping from her severed trachea through the pooling blood.

She continued to bleed, stopped breathing, and fell limp on the forest floor. "Coon" completed the decapitation by twisting the skull on the cervical spine until it came free. Horrified, Cody watched the whole killing, feeling he was unable to intervene on her behalf. Cody feared Coon would harm him as well. He became nauseated and vomited.

Coon cut a small wisp of hair from the scalp and placed it in his pocket. He told Cody the skull was worth $1,500 dollars to a buyer in Coeur d'Alene. Coon then had Cody help him drag the headless corpse up the hill, where they placed the body under a fallen log and covered it with brush and leaves. Coon wrapped the skull in Carissa's patterned sweater and stashed it in the crotch of a nearby tree. He discarded his bloody USS Nimitz tee shirt at the scene.

Coon told Cody he would kill him if he told anyone about the crime. He also indicated that Cody was now "eligible" to wear the Black Rose Tattoo.

*Back at the camp, Coon placed the bloody knife in the fire, and threw the blade into the brush. He also cut off the bloody cuffs of his jeans and burned them. Previously, he had burned Carissa's bra and swimsuit bottoms. They put out the fire, packed up the tent and sleeping bags, and headed back to Post Falls. They ditched the yellow Styrofoam cooler containing other camping items along the way. They also concocted an alibi to use when they got home.*

*One week later, Cody got his Black Rose Tattoo at the Lake City Tattoo parlor in Coeur d'Alene.*

*   *   *

*Detective Maskell and a small taskforce began accumulating evidence to present to Bill Douglas, the Kootenai County Prosecutor.*

*Meanwhile, Coon assaulted an acquaintance of Carissa Benway in his mobile home in Post Falls. He was arrested, convicted and sentenced to three to ten years in prison. He had served time previously in Washington State for child molestation.*

*Cody initially denied any involvement in the crime. He refused to implicate his father. He feared Coon would kill him, or have the "Brotherhood" kill him for snitching on a "Brother."*

*In subsequent interviews, Cody admitted he had witnessed Coon murder Carissa and had helped him dispose of the body. He said he got the Black Rose Tattoo at Lake City Tattoo. Maskell interviewed the tattoo shop owners. They confirmed that the Black Rose Tattoo was a gang sign and had a death connotation.*

*Detective Maskell obtained a search warrant for the Merritt mobile home. Detectives recovered several photos of Carissa Benway wearing the patterned sweater recovered at the crime scene. They also recovered a plastic box containing several wisps of hair. A neighbor said that Coon Merritt had frequently worn the "Nimitz" tee shirt, and kept it in the top drawer of a dresser at his home.*

*Kootenai County Sheriff Deputies arrested Cody Merritt in September 2001, and charged him with being an accessory to murder, rape and kidnapping. Detective Maskell brought Cody Merritt, under custody, to my office bearing a court order instructing me to obtain pubic and scalp hair samples, plus a cheek swab for DNA from Cody Merritt. I completed this in sterile conditions, under the role of my "doctor hat."*

*I placed the specimens in evidence envelopes, sealed them, and a chain-of-custody envelope was established. Detective Maskell witnessed the forms and submitted the evidence to the Idaho State Crime lab for comparison with hair samples found on the skeletal remains and the large piece of dried skin. In the face of possible prosecution for being an accessory to murder, kidnapping and rape, Cody Merritt agreed to provide testimony for the prosecution against his father.*

Kootenai County Sheriff arrested and charged David "Coon" Merritt on February 2nd, 2002. The Prosecutor charged him with kidnapping, rape and murder. At trial, he was convicted and sentenced to life in prison without parole. The Prosecutor arranged a plea bargain for Cody in return for testimony against his father. Cody Merritt received a reduced sentence.[5]

All of this happened in Kootenai County, Idaho. Amidst the beauty of our rolling hills and lakes, some very bad people still exist. Sometimes there are no outward signs to warn us. They prey on the young and old, rich or poor, local kids or transients. There is no one explanation for their behavior.

I agree that people can unwittingly, and willfully, place themselves in dangerous positions. Society will have to answer for allowing these criminals out on the street. We all need to be more vigilant when our kids begin skipping school, drinking alcohol, and using drugs, including marijuana. I personally believe both alcohol and marijuana are gateway drugs. I will deal with other drug problems in a later chapter.

My intent here is to outline the incredible amount of Forensic Science brought to bear in the Benway-Merritt case. The unrelenting efforts of Detective Maskell and a host of local and regional individuals helped solve this case and bring the perpetrators to justice. The sentinel

---

[5]    Coeur d'Alene Press, Feb. 1, 2001, "Benway's Mother Thankful" by Mike McLain and "Charges Filed in Benway Case" by Eric Flowers (excerpts used by permission.)

decision of the two hunters to bring in the jawbone essentially provided a key piece in the case. It also illustrates the how much we rely on the public for clues.

Skeletal Identification:

We are often called to various scenes in the county when unidentified skeletal remains are discovered. These may relate to Native American burials, private burials on old homestead sites, and a variety of other legitimate situations. Most of the time, such remains are of animals. Some animal skeletons (e.g. black bear) may have close similarity to human remains. The present Kootenai County Coroner has a Masters degree in Forensic Anthropology, in addition to her RN degree. The forensic anthropology departments at Eastern Washington University at Cheney, Washington and the Washington State Forensic Anthropologist have been of great assistance in resolving these cases.

*One Monday morning, I found an unusual, oblong, wooden case on the exam table at the Coroner's office. Dexter Yates, a local funeral home director gave me the background:*

*There are numerous fraternal organizations which flourished in many localities for years. Since WWII, there has been a gradual decline in membership in these organizations. Many have disbanded and closed their lodges and meeting places.*

*One such lodge in Post Falls disbanded several years ago. The women's auxiliary, however, remained active and housed paraphernalia of the parent lodge in a garage belonging to the mayor of Hayden Lake. As she and a friend were cleaning out the garage, they discovered this large oblong box. It had a "trapdoor" lid which, when opened, disclosed a skull and a fully articulated skeleton. They notified Yates Funeral Home who brought it to the Coroner's Office.*

*We examined the skeleton further and noted it was from a young adult female, on the basis of a gynecoid pelvis, non-erupted third molars, and a pubic symphysis that was not fused. The disposition of the skeleton was problematic. We determined that the skeleton was part of the Lodge's ceremonial activities. We contacted the national office of the organization.*

*They told us that in the 1920s, an Ohio anatomical supply company furnished numerous such skeletons to the organization for ceremonial use. With the disbandment of many of the lodges, a large number of the skeletons had ended up at the state and national offices. We arranged for the existing auxiliary unit make a formal donation of the skeleton to the Kootenai County Coroner's Office. The grounds caretaker at Coeur d'Alene Memorial Gardens fabricated an aluminum stand and "KC" now provides a forensic reference for our investigators to use in identification of skeletal remains.*

As with all such specimens, due respect is shown to the unknown donor. We are grateful to the lodge for the specimen.

As an aside, most anatomic supply catalogs now only have plastic reproductions of skeletons for such purposes. The prices range up to two thousand dollars. Actual skeletons from Asia are even more expensive.

# CHAPTER 10

# THE SUICIDE "EPIDEMIC"

Suicide is a very complex issue that coroners deal with on a regular basis. I recommend several helpful resources for a thorough examination of the suicide problem.[6]

Idaho has a relatively high rate-per-100,000 for suicide. This is especially troubling in the under-twenty age group. Society tends to avoid many of the issues associated with suicide. More than 50% of suicides are associated with alcohol. One common feature is an extreme feeling of distancing from family, and a loss of self-worth. I tend to disagree with Joiner regarding the issue of the aggressive nature of suicide toward those left behind. Nonetheless, coroners agonize over these cases.

*On May 30, 1976, our eldest son, Steve, was graduating from Coeur d'Alene High School. As a member of the Board of Trustees of School District #271, I was looking forward to awarding him his diploma.*

*About four o'clock in the afternoon, I was finishing my last outpatient when we received a phone call from a very distraught Mrs. Frank Reynolds. She explained that when she came home from work, a note on the table warned her not to come out to the barn where her husband's pickup was*

---

[6]    See T. J. Joiner's book, *Myths about Suicide* (Harvard University press, 2010); the suicide prevention courses by Paul Quinnette, PhD: *QPR—Question, Persuade, Refer;* and The Institute of Medicine study "Reducing Suicide: A National Imperative" (National Academies Press – 2002).

*parked. She described a half-empty gallon of Vodka on the table, along with several other empty liquor bottles along with the suicide note.*

*I told her to call the KCSO and that I would head out to their farm about ten miles from Coeur d'Alene. My teenage sons had swapped cars and left me with their 1964 Ford Fairlane with less than a quarter tank of gas. I headed out to Cougar Gulch promptly without breaking the speed limit. After all, most coroner cases are not an extreme emergency.*

*When I arrived at the Reynolds' farmhouse, Mrs. Reynolds met me at the door and showed me the note and the empty liquor bottles. I donned my "coroner hat" and proceeded out to the pickup. A body was slumped over in the passenger's side of the cab. As I looked into the vehicle, the victim suddenly moaned and moved. I could see a massive head wound. He was holding a .357-caliber revolver in his right hand. I went around to the passenger side of the truck, opened the door, and gingerly removed the gun from the victim's hand.*

*Ordinarily, I would have waited for the KCSO deputy to arrive and secure the weapon. I felt there was a greater risk he would discharge another round at himself or me.*

*Now, I was back in "doctor mode." I yelled for Mrs. Reynolds to call 911 for an ambulance to respond to the scene. She alerted them we had a severe head gunshot wound. We would need transport to Kootenai Medical Center and then to Sacred Heart Hospital in Spokane, since no Neurosurgeons were on staff at KMC in 1976.*

*The victim's airway was obstructed due to his position in the vehicle. While supporting his head and cervical spine, we removed him from the vehicle to a supine position on the ground until the ambulance arrived. They took over the care of the patient, started an IV, and transported him to KMC, and later to Sacred Heart Medical Center.*

*By this time, the KCSO deputy arrived. He interviewed Mrs. Reynolds and myself, and took possession of the weapon.*

*(I did make it to the graduation ceremony just before they got to the "Ws.")*

*Frank Reynolds survived the gunshot wound (GSW). He eventually had a titanium plate installed over the missing portion of his skull. The net result of the GSW was, essentially, a frontal lobotomy. He was a very pleasant individual with an insatiable appetite and developed extreme obesity. Otherwise, he was affable and showed no other aftereffects from the massive head wound. He also never again tried to commit suicide.*

Reynolds joined another patient of mine who survived his attempt to commit suicide by gunshot wound to the head.

*Carl Stoicheff, a depressed alcoholic, regularly consumed alcohol in vast quantities. After a long day of heavy drinking, Carl placed a .38-caliber pistol beneath his chin and pulled the trigger. The bullet went through the floor of his mouth, knocked off two upper incisors, took off a portion of his nasal bone, and exited through his frontal sinus. The bullet followed the midline almost perfectly.*

*I was the on-call surgeon when he came into the emergency room. We found fragments of teeth in his mouth, but the nasal bone fragments were missing. Aside from ecchymosis of both eyelids, there were no injuries to the bony orbits or contents. After several surgeries to repair various bony structures in his nose and frontal sinuses, he survived with little other damage.*

*Unfortunately, about three years later, I received a coroner call to his home in Post Falls. Mr. Stoicheff had committed suicide by slashing both brachial arteries and veins in the antecubital fossa with a razor. He bled into a garbage can placed at his bedside.*

The tragedy here is that ineffective efforts to treat his alcoholism and/or underlying psychiatric disorder after his first attempted suicide led to a completed suicide.

Persistent suicidal thoughts and feelings are markers for unremitting, unendurable psychological pain and suffering. Psychological pain is one term that covers distress, despair, depression, rage, anxiety, isolation or hopelessness. A federal survey in 2008 reported that in *one* year the adult American Psychological Pain index was as follows:

- 8.3 million of us seriously considered suicide
- 2.2 million of us made a plan to kill ourselves
- 1 million of us made an actual suicide attempt

In 2010, this pain contributed to 38,364 completed suicides in the United States. That is 105 Americans per day year after year. Can you imagine what Congress and the President would do if a commercial airliner loaded with one-hundred-plus passengers crashed every single day after day after day?

A CDC study in 2010 showed that six western states had suicide rates above 18/ 100,000. The Idaho rate is 18.5/100,000. Males are nearly four times more likely to commit suicide. The rate for Whites is greater than African-Americans, Asians or Hispanics.

There are approximately 1,200 total deaths a year in the in Kootenai County. We average thirty-five to forty suicides a year. There were 11,848 total deaths in Idaho in 2011. Idaho's population was 132,000 (2010 Census). What is lost in these numbers is the incredible toll this takes on individuals, their relatives and society in general. To date, efforts to address this issue have been minuscule at best. We tend to sublimate the issue, not addressing the reality of the suicide. When today's headline is past, the family is left with an empty hole that desperately needs filling. Survivor groups only begin to touch the problem without grasping the societal impact of suicide.

We truly need to implement a national and local strategy for reducing suicide. The United States Air Force published a multi-year study in the *British Medical Journal*[7] clearly demonstrating that a robust, mandatory, suicide prevention/mental health promotion program dramatically reduced violence of all kinds. Their findings:

- 33% drop in suicides
- 18% drop in homicides
- 54% drop in serious family violence
- 30% drop in moderate family violence
- 18% drop in accidental deaths (some of which were likely disguised suicides)

The Veteran's Administration is implementing a proactive program of suicide prevention, particularly in veterans returning from the wars

---

[7]   Knox, K.L., Litts, D.A., Talcott. G.W., Feig. J.C., Caine, E.D., 2003: *Risk of Suicide and related adverse outcomes after exposure to a suicide prevention programme in the U.S. Air Force, cohort study:* British Medical Journal, 13.327.(7428)

in Iraq and Afghanistan. The diagnoses of Post-Traumatic Stress Disorder (PTSD) and the related Post-Traumatic Stress Syndrome (PTSS) encompasses a whole range of patients, and probably overlooks a substantial number who are at risk for attempted/completed suicide.

*I saw this anguish in the case of a veteran who committed suicide by lighting a charcoal grill in his tool shed in the backyard. The deadly carbon monoxide bonded to his hemoglobin, suffocating him in minutes. Several cans of beer floated in an ice-filled basin on the floor. A photo of his wife in a broken picture frame lay next to the body, along with other mementos of a failed marriage. The aura of his psychological pain was palpable in that shed.*

Many other suicides offer a poignant picture of the extreme isolation of the victims as they proceed to end their lives. Someone once said, "Suicide is a permanent solution to a temporary problem." We cannot always predict the "tipping point," which pushes a person over the edge. We can be aware of some of the signs of depression, expressions of suicidal thoughts, or disposing of personal items, etc. Physicians, family and the general public should always be alert to warning signs and utilize the Question, Persuade, and Refer (QPR), method mentioned in the resources above.

A variety of materials are used as cervical ligatures in suicide cases. Belts, dog leashes, electrical cords, scarves, neckties, and of course, rope material have all been used. I cannot remember a single case with a so-called "hangman's noose." Most result in asphyxiation, rather than the cervical fracture and spinal cord transaction seen in criminal execution cases. We find most suicide victims shortly after death. Forensic investigation is frequently hampered when family members or emergency responders/law enforcers move the victim, displace the cervical ligature, or take the lifeless victim to the nearest medical facility.

*During the late spring run-off season, a woman walking her dog at the former Atlas Lumber Mill site on the Spokane River discovered a body suspended from a tree on the banks of the swollen river. Access to the area was treacherous due to an unstable riverbank and cold, river water. We cut the tree branch with the ligature material in place and carefully moved the body to a safe location. The body was partially mummified from exposure to* the cold, dry winter air for five months. The skin was leathery and showed little decomposition except for myriad insect eggs on the exposed mucous membranes. Crows had attacked the orbits and contents.

His wife had reported him missing in late January. He had just secured a position with a local Call Center after months of unemployment. He never showed up for work. We confirmed his identification by matching his driver's license photos and a Cd'A Police photo of his tattoos.

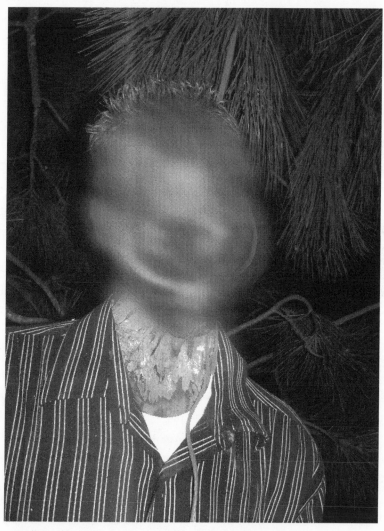

"Hanging Victim partially mummified after exposure
to dry, cold winter air for 5 months."

*A clinical psychologist from Kootenai Medical Center went missing in the Meadowbrook area south of Coeur d'Alene. Search parties with cadaver dogs spent several days in early September searching for the doctor. We searched his home, outbuildings and barn without finding the body. When the leaves fell in October, we found him hanging in a tree near one of the buildings. Curiously, his pager was on his belt along with other personal effects. We were unable to recover received pages from the device.*

*A KMC Staff Psychiatrist committed suicide in his office on Ironwood Drive. We found a .22-caliber revolver found next to the body. Inspection of his office records revealed illegal narcotic self-prescribing, plus a record of an on-going investigation by the Idaho State Board of Medicine and the Board of Pharmacy.*

It is important for family members to have an accurate assessment of their risk factors for any given disease. It is a fallacy to "assume" that a family history of a disease translates into the cause of death.

*The physician father of a local family of doctors and dentists died at age 45 from a massive coronary thrombosis. We found his dentist son deceased of unknown cause. Based on the family history, cardiovascular disease was suspected. Further investigation revealed that the dentist's physician recently told him he had Parkinson's disease. The tremors associated with Parkinson's disease would have detrimentally impacted his ability to practice dentistry. His toxicology results showed a lethal level of Oxycontin. There was minimal coronary atherosclerosis.*

*Another unusual case involved an employee of a compressed medical gas company in Spokane. He developed chronic back pain while delivering full-sized tanks of oxygen, nitrous oxide (laughing gas), and a variety of other gases to hospitals, medical and dental offices in Coeur d'Alene and Spokane. He had been placed on medical disability.*

*He resided in an apartment in the basement of his parent's home. His mother found him deceased with a plastic garbage sack tied around his neck with tubing attached to a nitrous oxide tank with the valve open. She removed the garbage sack, turned off the gas and called 911. She also shut down his computer monitor, which displayed many pornographic images.*

    *Nitrous oxide mixed with oxygen in a ratio of 85:15% is used as an anesthetic by doctors and dentists. However, at 100% concentration, it produces lethal hypoxia. We found a variety of other anesthetic gas tanks in his apartment and several full Vodka bottles. There were many assorted pornographic magazines and photos throughout the apartment. The Coeur d'Alene Police investigator seized the computer and other materials into evidence. For whatever reason, the police department did not have a forensic investigator search the hard drive for criminal evidence or victims of illicit sexual behavior.*

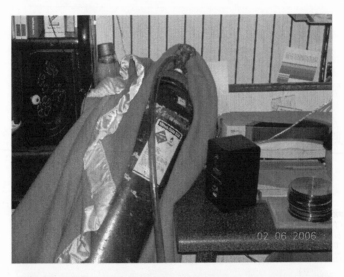

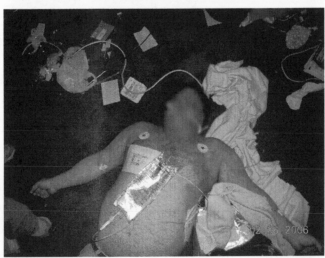

Nitrous Oxide victim with tubing and plastic sack

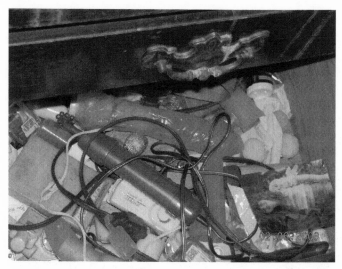

"Sex Toys"

The medical gas company retrieved their purloined tanks. We were not able to determine how this "disabled" man was able to haul a large tank of nitrous oxide downstairs to the basement without his parents being aware. It appeared that he was using the gas as an erotic stimulant while viewing pornography.

## Murder/Suicides

The majority of murder/suicide cases involve handguns and alcohol. Domestic disputes factor into the assessment of causation and intent. Many of the victims are elderly and/or disabled. A caregiver may reach a breaking point and act out of compassion, distress, or at the request of the murder victim. There are seldom notes defining intent although relatives may have had indications of intent.

*A husband returned to his Hayden Lake home after a night of drinking in a Quonset building he used as a shop. An argument ensued and both victims exchanged multiple gunshots. The wife had a .38-caliber revolver and a concealed weapons permit. The husband had a 9mm semi-automatic handgun.*

*When I arrived for the coroner investigation, the wife was deceased. Paramedics transported the husband to KMC where he later died. The investigating officers used laser pointers to ascertain the direction of fire of the various bullets. A deputy escorted me out to the shop where a loaded sawed off, 12-gauge shotgun was mounted in a vise directed at the door. They unloaded the gun but it was a reminder not to go charging around a crime scene until law enforcement has secured all weapons and/or other devices.*

\*     \*     \*

*In another poignant case, an elderly diabetic male picked up his wife at a local Nursing home expressing his desire to take her for a drive around Coeur d'Alene. She had been complaining of "bronchitis" for several days but seemed excited about the extra activity.*

*When they did not return to the nursing home by 8 p.m., the nursing home staff became concerned and notified the family. The family responded to the residence where both the husband and wife were found deceased in the living room. There were several partially empty vials of insulin in the refrigerator prescribed for the husband's diabetes. Two used insulin syringes were on the kitchen counter.*

*Our initial impression was of a murder/suicide due to deliberate insulin overdose. However, postmortem blood cultures from the wife disclosed overwhelming sepsis due to Hemophilus Influenzae and a normal blood glucose level. The husband's post-mortem blood sugar was less than 30 mg% which was consistent with hyper-insulinemia. Therefore, the wife's death was classified as "natural" due to H. Influenzae infection. The husband's death was classified as due to hyper-insulinemia with hypo-glycemia (low blood sugar). The manner was listed as "could not be determined." There was only circumstantial evidence of intent.*

The lesson here is that a correct diagnosis is important both from the vital statistics standpoint but also for the surviving family members. As indicated above, death certificates are confidential for 100 years in Idaho. The coroner cannot "assume" that the manner of death is either suicide or homicide without proof.

\*     \*     \*

*Spokane County Sheriff and Kootenai County Sheriff Deputies were pursuing a convicted felon in a stolen vehicle eastbound on I-90 west of Post Falls. The felon ditched the car near Corbin Park, exited the vehicle and jumped into the Spokane River which was running at winter flows of approximately 3,000 cubic feet per second. He never emerged on the opposite shore. He was presumed drowned with associated immersion hypothermia.*

*In late spring, we found his body entangled in trees on the banks of the Spokane River just east of the Washington border. He had the keys from the stolen vehicle in his pocket. The felon had multiple distinguishing tattoos, which matched those on booking photos Washington authorities provided to the Coroner's Office. Prophetically, one tattoo indicated where to place his toe tag.*

*We were unable to certify the identification of the body in time to prevent a Spokane bail bondsman from losing a $40,000 bail bond he had posted before our victim stole the car. We had to make certain we had the correct identification before issuing a death certificate, listing the case as an accidental drowning.*

*If the body had been located a few hundred feet further west, the case would have come under the jurisdiction of Spokane County.*

\*     \*     \*

*We found skeletal remains and a revolver in a wooded area near Hayden Lake. We made the identification by means of an esophageal speech device near the skeleton. We matched the serial and model numbers of the device and the revolver to the victim.*

*Several years previously, the victim had undergone a laryngectomy and radiation therapy for cancer of the vocal cords. Speech therapy using the artificial voice box was satisfactory. He had no evidence of recurrent or distant disease and was declared cancer-free.*

*His live-in girlfriend developed a relationship with another male, which only added to his depression over his medical condition. He felt unwelcome in the home when the other male displaced him. He went into the woods in November and, despite an extensive search, the skeletal remains were not found until the snow melted in the spring.*

*     *     *

Another case involved two Asian exchange students, attending a college in Spokane, went for a drive in the area south of Blossom Mountain on the Washington/Idaho border. They turned north off Elder Road and proceeded up into the foothills. The snowpack had melted and the roads were extremely muddy. The area provides few places where you can turn around. Somehow, they and another car became mired in a large mud hole. Neither vehicle could be extricated from it. They spent the night in their respective cars.

When daylight came, the students found the driver of the other car deceased. The driver had attached a hose to the exhaust pipe of his car and placed it in a rear window. His car license matched that of a vehicle involved in a shootout with police in Cheney, WA on the day before his discovery in Idaho. The driver had fled the scene, avoiding police pursuit. He ended up in the foothills area, and killed himself by attaching a hose to the exhaust pipe of his car and placing it in a side window.

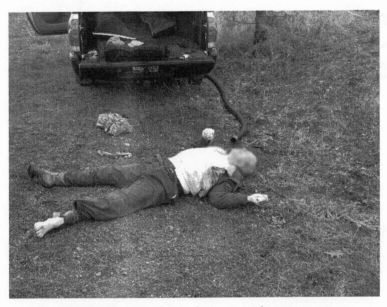

Victim placed exhaust hose in pickup canopy

# Hospital Homicides

*An intensive care unit nurse at the Kootenai Medical Center heard a gunshot in one of the patient rooms. She discovered a critically ill ventilator patient had been shot by a distraught relative to "put her out of her misery." The weapon was recovered and the relative charged with manslaughter.*

Protecting hospital patients and staff from assaults by guns and other weapons has been partially successful with implementation of increased security, surveillance and secure key-lock entry systems.

Security of pharmacy carts and automated record of access and medications dispensation are only partially successful in preventing accidental and/or deliberate injury to patients. Recent legislation passed by the Idaho legislature now makes it a felony to assault a health care worker unless under the influence of a prescribed medication. The bill awaits the signature of the Governor.

# Munchausen Syndrome and Munchausen-by-proxy

Baron Munchausen was a German nobleman working in the Russian army who fabricated impossible stories of wide travels. In 1951, Richard Asher named this syndrome of self-inflicted harm, multiple unnecessary hospitalizations, operations and occasional loss of life.

Munchausen-by-proxy is a form of child abuse, which involves the exaggeration or fabrication of illnesses or symptoms by a primary caretaker, and is an uncommon occurrence in hospitalized patients.

*I cared for a male patient presented to KMC with bleeding and an extremely prolonged prothrombin time. He was not on any known coumadin derivatives. However, blood tests showed coumadin breakdown products. We administered Vitamin K and fresh frozen plasma to reverse the abnormal clotting time and eventually brought his prothrombin times back to normal. Following discharge, he again developed the symptoms and we eventually discovered that his wife was placing D-Con in his food.*

Note: Coumadin (Warfarin) was discovered by researchers at the University of Wisconsin Alumni Research Foundation in 1948, hence the acronym. It is still used as a pesticide in rat poison. Approved by the FDA in 1954, the patent proceeds from Warfarin and its derivatives have funded large portions of the budget at the University of Wisconsin for years. Coumadin is the most widely prescribed anticoagulant in the United States.

*An example of Munchausen by proxy involved the illicit introduction of foreign material in intravenous solutions was suspected in a child who ran fevers of unknown origin. Monitored surveillance of the patient eventually identified the mother as the source of the material. She was committed for mental evaluation.*

## Russian Roulette

This is an interesting subset of suicides which has engendered much discussion in recent years. Some experts say these should be classified as "accidental," since there seldom is a prior expression of intent. The frequent associations of alcohol intoxication and peer-group pressures are factors in these discussions.

Other experts suggest that these victims make the following six discrete, conscious decisions:

1.  Obtains or has access to a gun. (revolver or other handgun.)
2.  Places a round in the cylinder.
3.  Closes the cylinder.
4.  Cocks the hammer.
5.  Places the barrel of the revolver against his skull or in his mouth.
6.  Spins the cylinder while pulling the trigger.

By making these decisions, the victim has reduced the odds of being shot in the head from approximately infinity to one in six. Further reduction of these odds may result when the victim pulls the trigger *more* than once. There are several reports of such attempts both fatal and nonfatal.

Other fatal episodes occur when the victim does not account for the clockwise vs. counter-clockwise rotation of the cylinder. In Colt revolvers the cylinder rotates clockwise, whereas, in Smith & Wesson revolvers the cylinder rotates counter-clockwise.

Incidentally, these same six decisions are made when the actions involve two or more people, in which case it is a homicide.

*One victim had a habit of "miming" by pointing his index finger to his temple and mock firing whenever he was distressed or on the losing side of some argument. On the day of his death, he became embroiled with an employee over a payroll matter. He reached into a desk drawer, pulled out his revolver, placed the barrel to his temple and pulled the trigger. The result was instantly fatal. Despite his history of "simulated" firings, the fact is that he voluntarily completed all six of the steps outlined above for "Russian Roulette."*

I am too much of a Clint Eastwood fan to endorse the draconian penalties assessed on schoolchildren for similar miming activities. The "PC Police" should explore other behavioral methods rather than resorting to school expulsion or prosecution.

It is often difficult to differentiate between "accidental" deaths and "intentional" suicides. Many factors must be considered before one makes the final distinction. Families are counseled that while the coroner may have reached a conclusion that a given death is the result of suicide, they are under no responsibility to disclose the cause or manner of death to the public, the media, or any other persons.

Death certificates in Idaho remain confidential and subject to Federal HIPPA regulations for one hundred years from the date of death.

The death certificate or autopsy reports may only be released to the Next of Kin. Each state has a distinct order of priority for next-of-kin determination. In Idaho, it does *not* include an ex-spouse, common law spouse, domestic partner, or several others. On the other hand, persons separated but still married retain their next-of-kin status. The next of kin *may* decide to release the death certificate or autopsy report to other persons. (Note: It will be interesting to see how this Next-of-Kin issue plays out in cases where an Out-of-State legal same-sex marriage has one person die and the determination of Next-of-Kin falls to the coroner or the mortician.)

*We found a young man hanged on Tubbs Hill, a popular park in downtown Coeur d'Alene. There were no other signs of external injury. The autopsy was consistent with asphyxiation due to cervical ligature. His toxicology was negative, although there was an unsubstantiated history of "pot" smoking with his friends prior to his death.*

*The family was adamant that he had been murdered and the body moved to Tubbs Hill, and the rope placed post-mortem to "appear" like suicide. This controversy continued for several years until the family obtained a court order for disinterment and a second autopsy. The results of that autopsy were similar to the first. The cause and manner of death remain unchanged.*

*In another case, however, we were able to determine a different cause and manner of death. A female (G.D.) North Idaho College student was at an off-campus party where there was alcohol in abundance, as well as illicit drugs. She obtained what she believed was "LSD" from a male at the party. Shortly after ingesting the material, she became delirious and unconscious. They brought her to Kootenai Medical Center Emergency Room. Her temperature soared to 105–107 degrees. She developed seizures and shortly succumbed without ever regaining consciousness.*

*The KMC toxicology screen showed only an elevated blood alcohol level of 0.1gm% and no LSD metabolites. We submitted serum and urine samples to the Miami-Dade County Medical Examiner-Toxicology Division. Although it took them fourteen months to complete the testing, they reported the presence of the so-called "Designer Drug" (5-Methoxy-alpha-methyl-tryptamine), which has a profile of side effects exactly mirroring our case.*

*We reclassified the case as a homicide due to drug toxicity. The "doper" who provided the substance to her was convicted of manslaughter and given a prison sentence.*

We are often criticized for the dollar costs of toxicology testing. The modern spectrum of therapeutic and illicit drugs is simply beyond the scope of local/regional labs. As the 'ombudsman' for the deceased, I feel strongly that a decision to search out the true cause of death is vitally important. Not every case can or should be subjected to this level of scrutiny. Fiscal and time constraints weigh into these decisions. We recognize some cases are bound to slip by without timely investigation. However, each case deserves and receives careful consideration before being signed out. Every coroner struggles to sort out each case on its own merits and make the best decision with the knowledge at hand.

# CHAPTER 11

# PIMPS, PROSTITUTES AND JOHNS

Like many western states, Idaho has a long and colorful history of hell-roaring mining towns with saloons, gambling, and the ever-present brothels and purveyors of the "world's oldest profession." During the construction of the Milwaukee Railroad Hiawatha Route through the Bitteroot Mountains in 1908–1910, saloons and brothels outnumbered boarding houses. Several of the "madams" who ran brothels in the Silver Valley acquired notoriety for their community service on behalf of the "girls." Whether deserved or not, the sad fact is that sex trafficking remains one of the seamier sides of civilization, even today. Not just in the developing third world countries of Southeast Asia or Sub-Saharan Africa, but here in the Inland Northwest, including Kootenai County. Active prostitution rings still recruit or kidnap girls as young as thirteen to service customers at major events such as the Super Bowl and other large conventions.

In their 2009 book, *Half the Sky*, Nicholas Kristof and Sheryl Wu Dunn[8] extensively document sex trafficking around the world, and offer suggestions for combating it.

---

[8] Kristoff, Nicholas and WuDunn, Sheryl, "Half the Sky," Alfred E. Knopf, New York, 2009

*Between 1996 and 1998, William H. Yates murdered at least thirteen women in Spokane, Washington. Most were prostitutes and drug users. The anonymous nature of those women's lives, their pimps, and the "Johns" who frequented them, made them easy targets for a serial killer.*

*As far as is known, none of the GPS waypoints programmed into the Magellan 2000 GPS unit found in Yates' house pinpoint locations in Kootenai County. He even buried one body beneath his bedroom window.*

*Yates was an Air National Guard helicopter pilot in Spokane. He was also stationed at Ft. Lewis- McCord base in Tacoma, Washington and he deployed to Germany with the Washington Air National Guard.*

*He is currently serving a 448-year sentence in Washington State, and has a number of other convictions including a death sentence for a murder in western Washington. German authorities consider him a person of interest in several murders occurring during his deployment in Germany with the United States Air Force.*

That this killer operated at random for three years fewer than thirty miles from Coeur d'Alene is both chilling and daunting. The dehumanizing effect on prostitutes, and society's marginalization of them, leads to many of the crimes associated with these women.

*A Spokane pimp invited his troupe of prostitutes to a weekend cocaine party at Hauser Lake in Kootenai County. He brought along a "brick" of cocaine that he provided to his drug-addicted prostitutes. One prostitute, in her twenties, stole his car and the stash of cocaine. She drove around Kootenai County shooting up with cocaine and other drugs. The Post Falls Police found her nude body along the railway tracks in Post Falls with a syringe still in her antecubital vein. They discovered pornographic magazines and photographs in the car's trunk plus other drug paraphernalia. The police impounded the car and later returned it to the pimp. The question remains whether she self-overdosed on cocaine, or whether the pimp found her and administered a fatal "hot shot."*

*Even though we discovered the body within hours of her death, "Blow Flies" (**Musca Carnaria**) had already zoned in on the dead body. They had deposited myriad eggs on her eyelids, nostrils and mucous membranes.*

*Researchers have shown that a female blow fly can detect a dead body for up to a mile, and will make a beeline to deposit her eggs. In the hot August weather, the body would have been transformed into a teaming mass of maggots within days.*

Prostitution does not deserve the label of "victimless crime!"

\*    \*    \*

*A hysterical, naked woman appeared at the door of a home on Hayden Creek Road early on a May morning. Residents took her inside, wrapped her in a blanket and called 911. Paramedics and KCSO deputies responded to the scene. The paramedics bandaged her wounds and transported her to Kootenai Medical Center where surgeons repaired the wounds. She bore defensive knife wounds on both arms and hands. Toxicology revealed metabolites of cocaine and methamphetamine.*

*The Coeur d'Alene Police interviewed her in the hospital. She told Coeur d'Alene Police she was working in Spokane's First Avenue red-light district as a prostitute. She admitted using cocaine and methamphetamine shortly before being picked up by the "John." The stranger in a pickup stopped and asked her to perform oral sex. She told him her price for a "trick" was fifty dollars. However, he offered her $300 for an "all-night stand." She agreed and got in the truck.*

*He began driving around Spokane and eventually over to Kootenai County. He drove around Hayden Lake and turned up Hayden Creek Road, still covered with about six to eight inches of packed snow and ice. They came to a deserted borrow-pit, which local hunters use as a makeshift shooting range. He parked the truck, held her at knifepoint and raped her. He also told her he had raped and killed twelve other women and disposed of their bodies in the Coeur d'Alene National Forest.*

*Somehow, she managed to grab the knife from the rapist and inflict multiple stab wounds to his neck and head until he died. She left him in a pool of blood and snowmelt. She threw the folding knife in a puddle of water, and took his truck.*

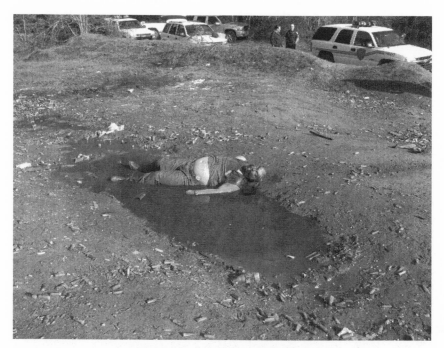

"Murdered Rapist in Puddle."

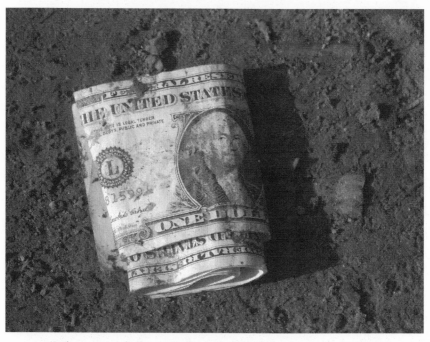

"Three one dollar bills found at Hayden murder scene."

Initially, she drove further up Hayden Creek road but eventually turned the truck around, drove back past the borrow-pit and stopped at the Hayden Creek residence.

The physicians at KMC emergency department admitted her for observation because of the drug screen results and her mental status. The Women's Center eventually housed her in a local motel until she returned to Spokane, Washington.

Meanwhile, KCSO deputies impounded the truck for evidence. They proceeded up Hayden Creek road about a mile and a half to the borrow-pit where they found the body and other evidence.

Deputy Coroner Deb Wilkey and I navigated the treacherous, icy road by four-wheel drive SUV to the site. KCSO Investigators showed us a body lying in a pool of blood and water. There were three one-dollar bills lying in a smaller pool of water along with a closed folding blade knife. The victim had extensive head and neck lacerations. His trousers were buttoned and secured by a large cowboy belt and buckle at the waist. He was wearing cowboy boots with the trousers tucked in the boots. Literally thousands of empty shotgun and rifle cartridges cluttered the borrow-pit.

It would have taken a task force a month to sort the empty cartridges, had this been a shooting death!

The KCSO investigators and Coroner took multiple measurements, and photographs of the scene and the truck-tire tracks. Due to the treacherous road conditions and the non-availability of a suitable funeral home vehicle, I placed the tagged body in a sealed body bag with the hands secured with paper bags in my SUV and transported it to the Spokane Medical Examiners facility. We stopped at the Coroner's Office to enter the information into the Med-Track system and submit an autopsy request. We then drove to the SCME autopsy facility.

Two KCSO deputies met us there to observe the autopsy, performed by Sally Aiken, M.D., the Spokane County Medical Examiner. Notably, the victim had nearly one hundred stab wounds, including several severing his carotid arteries and jugular veins. His bladder contained more than 1,000cc of urine. His lower legs showed muscular atrophy and deformity. He sustained no mutilation of his genitals or abdominal stab wounds. Examination of clothing and the genital regions disclosed no seminal fluid.

*The Medical Examiner took DNA samples from the genitalia, fingernails and buccal mucosa.*

*Medical history obtained from family members indicated that the victim suffered from a congenital neurologic disorder of the lower extremities making it difficult for him to walk.*

*The Kootenai County Prosecutor and Sheriff's office ruled the case a justifiable homicide based on self-defense. The prostitute was never charged. We later learned she had several prior assault charges in Spokane, including a knife attack involving her brother.*

This case was troubling and difficult. Many questions lie outside the purview of the Coroner's Office. It does illustrate some of the attitudes the public holds against certain segments of the population. Whether "he had it coming" or not, the fact remains that a human being was murdered. I cannot speak to the significance of the three, one-dollar bills in relation to the agreed upon price for an "all-night" stand.

It does bring to mind the 2003 movie, *Monster* in which Charlize Theron portrayed a Florida prostitute and serial killer who murdered several of her clients over a thirteen-month period.

We never found any evidence of other victims' bodies disposed of in the National Forest. Remember, however, there are more than one million acres in the Panhandle National Forest stretching from Coeur d'Alene to the Montana border. The "John's" familiarity with the Hayden Creek road in the middle of the night does raise the possibility of prior experience on that road.

# CHAPTER 12

# THE ENVIRONMENT IS ALWAYS AROUND US

North Idaho and the Rathdrum Prairie have an ideal climate and topography for the cultivation of bluegrass seed used in lawns and golf courses around the world. Thousands of acres of bluegrass fields stretch from Sandpoint to Plummer, Idaho, and into Washington State. Plentiful water for irrigation is necessary for the bluegrass to mature. Massive combines thresh the seeds, which are then transported to processing facilities.

The Jacklin Seed Company sorts, separates, and stores thousands of tons of bluegrass seed at its plant in Post Falls. This is marketed worldwide to consumers, including golf courses and homeowners.

One of the cultivation methods used to ensure a vigorous fall growth of the plants is to burn the stubble fields in the fall. This stimulates the plants to send down root systems, which then produce more and better seed the following season. The process also eliminates noxious weed seeds in the bluegrass fields.

The field burning in August and September uses a meteorological forecast of temperatures and wind conditions to allow the grass farmers to set thousands of acres of bluegrass stubble aflame. Smoke billowing to several thousand feet is a startling sight in country where most smoke can only mean one thing: forest fires. For the majority of field burning, the forecasts on burn days have allowed the smoke to dissipate away from population centers with minimal disruption in people's daily lives.

In other cases, an inversion holds the cloud of smoke at the surface, producing a choking, throat burning irritating environment, which can produce severe symptoms, especially in persons with respiratory diseases such as asthma or chronic obstructive pulmonary disease. These patients are told to stay indoors and avoid excessive exposure to the smoke. Clean Air advocates began to agitate against the field burning in the late 1970s. They formed an advocacy group, SAFE (Safe Air for Everyone,) to focus their efforts and produce changes in the tilling methods.

*M.M. was a breast cancer survivor patient of mine who worked as a waitress in Rathdrum. We had to manage her asthma very carefully during her surgery and recovery. My medical colleagues managed her asthma and were of great help in that respect. As the field-burning season approached, M.M would frequently call to have her asthma medications filled or her home nebulizer refilled.*

*One evening after the day's field burning had subsided, a pall of smoke descended over Rathdrum, restricting visibility for drivers and causing severe symptoms to many patients. M.M stayed indoors and did not show up for her waitress job. She developed respiratory distress in the early evening hours. She called 911, and an ambulance was dispatched to her home. When they arrived, M.M. was deceased on a couch in the living room. Her nebulizer was still running and other asthma medications sat on a table near her. The paramedics were unable to resuscitate her.*

*At autopsy, her lungs were hyperaerated, extending across the midline from both thoracic cavities. The bronchiospasm induced by the air pollution prevented air from being exhaled and the lungs became hyper-inflated. This produced progressive hypoxia and eventually caused her death. The immediate cause of death was "acute asthmatic hypoxic death," due to "severe environmental pollution," due to "grass field burning."*

There was a huge outcry over the Coroner blaming the field burning for M.M.'s death. The particle count on that day was in the thousands. I received numerous angry calls from grass farmers and industry representatives stating that I was destroying their ability to farm profitably.

It reminded me of the vilification physicians received from the tobacco industry when they began coding lung cancer deaths as due to "chronic exposure to tobacco." The Surgeon General's landmark "Report on Smoking and Health[9]" was published in 1964. The subsequent publication of large-scale, double-blind studies clearly identified tobacco smoke and other tobacco products as the underlying cause of the majority of lung cancer deaths, as well as many other public health problems.

SAFE filed a class-action lawsuit against the bluegrass growers. The suit was successful, and several plaintiffs received compensation from the seed growers. The farmers converted to a "no-till" method. The field burning has been discontinued on the Rathdrum Prairie, although the Coeur d'Alene Tribe south of Plummer still burns their grass fields. Therefore, we still have to contend with a smoke problem, but to a lesser extent.

I believe, then as now, the cause and manner of death determination was correct. There certainly was no conscious effort to impugn actions of any specific group or persons. *U.S. News and World Report* picked up the story and ran a feature detailing the noxious effects of field burning and my actions in declaring the cause of death.

Crops raised on the Rathdrum prairie require irrigation from deep well water in the aquifer. Many young people were hired by farmers to change irrigation pipes on a twelve-hour cycle during the growing season. Thirty-foot sections of aluminum piping must be disconnected from the supply source, the water in the section drained and moved to the successive strip of alfalfa or other crop. It is hard work and usually two or more people work in concert to speed up the process.

---

[9]    "Smoking and Health: Report of the Advisory Committee to the Surgeon General CDC" 1964

*Two young men were changing irrigation pipes. One of them raised a section of pipe vertically and contacted an overhead power line, which electrocuted him instantly. We responded to the scene and documented the proximity of the power line to the irrigation pipes. Most manual pipe-changing operations have been replaced by large mechanized circle or linear irrigation equipment to reduce such accidents and to provide an even level of water to thirsty crops.*

One of the continuing legacies of the mining industry in the Silver Valley is the lead and heavy metal contamination in the environment downstream from the mines and smelter. Vegetation in the Silver Valley was destroyed by the sulfur dioxide emanating from the Bunker Hill smelter's smokestack. Runoff from abandoned mines along the course of the East Fork of the Coeur d'Alene River rendered it very contaminated and devoid of any fish.

Installation of sewage treatment and heavy metal containment has restored the fishery and much of the natural environment. Following the dismantling of the Bunker Hill smelter in 1996, thousands of trees have been replanted and the forest is beginning to regrow. Lead and other heavy metal contamination resulted in the Environmental Protection Administration (EPA) declaring a superfund cleanup site called "The Box" in the Silver Valley from Mullan, Idaho to Lake Coeur d'Alene. Contractors have removed thousands of cubic yards of topsoil from yards and playgrounds and transported it to a repository where it is capped to prevent further contamination of the environment. Topsoil from out of the area has been brought in to replace the coverage in yards and playgrounds.

Along the old railway bed from Mullan to Plummer, lead- and zinc-contaminated soil has been capped and paved making the beautiful "Trail of the Coeur d'Alenes" bike and hiking trail, one of the premier attractions in North Idaho. Thousands of hikers and bikers use the trail each year.

However, during high run-off periods, such as a winter rain-on-snow event, or rapid spring snowmelt, hundreds of tons of soil containing heavy metal contaminants are "flushed" down the Coeur d'Alene River and into Lake Coeur d'Alene. Most of the lead, cadmium, zinc and other heavy metals remain as inert salts on the lake bottom. When disturbed or oxidized by the process of eutrophication, they represent a hazard to wildlife and humans.

Migrating Tundra Swans and Canada Geese have died after ingesting lead shotgun pellets while feeding on vegetation in the chain lakes bordering the Coeur d'Alene River. The neurologic sequelae of the lead render them unable to eat or fly. The bird carcasses contain high levels of lead. Other sources are leaded fishing weights and tire-balancing weights. Leaded gasoline is no longer sold in the United States for the same reasons.

Children with elevated blood lead levels exhibit diminished neurologic function and intellectual capacity. Most of these problems represent long-term effects, but also impact death investigation. The Panhandle Health District has a long-range project measuring lead levels in children in the Silver Valley.

The EPA has not always enjoyed a collaborative relationship with the mining industry, businesses, and public in the Silver Valley. The remediation results have shown significant decreases in the serum lead levels in children in the Silver Valley. The Panhandle Health district continues to monitor the children.

My relationship with the EPA evolved further from another interesting incident in Kootenai County.

*On a Friday night in September, Hauser Lake and Kootenai Fire Units responded to a mobile home fire near Rathdrum, Idaho. A KCSO deputy notified me around midnight and asked me to respond to the scene. First responders reported a body inside the burning mobile home. When I arrived, the fire crews were still battling an active fire. It was clear that no entry to the home would be possible until the site had cooled down.*

*Firefighters moved ten twenty-five-pound propane tanks from the porch to the lawn where another twenty similar sized tanks were strewn. Two tanks exploded in the mobile home while the fire was at its peak. Crews from Avista Utilities shut off a natural gas line to the mobile home. Firefighters felt the scene was too hot and unstable for entry. We secured the scene overnight while fire crews maintained one engine and crew to control any rekindling of the fire. The Idaho fire marshal investigator,*

*KCSO deputies and I agreed to return at daylight to proceed with the investigation.*

*Next morning, the death investigation team cautiously approached the smoldering ruins. We did not know whether we would find other unexploded tanks in the burned out rubble. They removed a portion of the exterior wall of the mobile home to access the living room, where we found the charred body. We secured the remains and sent them to the Spokane Medical Examiner for autopsy. Dental records confirmed the identification of Gary Lindgren, CEO of Oz Technologies.*

*None of the tanks in the yard of the home had EPA-approved overflow valves. Oz Technology would buy truckloads of the outmoded tanks from an unknown supplier and use them as reservoirs for the business. Oz Technology's business consisted of producing 6-oz. canisters containing a mixture of 49% butane and 51% propane.*

*Lingren marketed the mixture to air conditioning retailers under the labels HC12a and HC22 as a replacement for the hydroflurocarbon (HFC134 Freon) refrigerants outlawed in 1996 by the Montreal Protocols on Ozone Depletion. Lindgren obtained a US Patent (Patent # 6,336,333 B1) for the mixture in January 2002. He also claimed United Kingdom and Mexican patents with a distribution network around the United States. His Web site advertised the 6-oz. containers, plus 25-lb. and 50-lb. containers. The Web site extolled the virtues of this "new" product. The Consumer Product Safety Commission denied his application to market the product due to safety concerns. This did not constrain him from purchasing large quantities of propane and butane and mass-producing the canisters.*

*One outbuilding contained bulk propane and butane tanks, plus gas metering equipment. Another building housed palletized cartons of the 6-oz. canisters bearing the HC12a and HC22 labels, ready for shipment.*

*My Coroner duties were officially over when the autopsy results came back and we signed out the death certificate with "thermal conflagration" as the cause of death, and "accidental" as the manner of death. The following Tuesday, I contacted the battalion chief from the Hauser Lake Fire District to ask about the disposition of the remainder of the propane/butane tanks and the palletized containers. He indicated that the scene was going to be released to the "probable responsible party" (PRP). I asked who that might be, and he did not know. They were still trying to locate Lindgren's next of kin.*

*The Oz Technology bookkeeper arrived at the scene while we were extricating the body. She confirmed there was an active ongoing business. However, she had no legal standing to arrange disposition of the materials.*

The scene was potentially the most dangerous I ever encountered in forty-one years as Coroner. The grass grew waist high and was extremely dry in late summer. The mobile home was located in a wooded area with numerous homes within a mile. The slopes of nearby ridges were forested and equally dry. In short, the ingredients for a major firestorm lay in wait with literally thousands of leaking canisters of this flammable mixture. I understood that local law and fire agencies were interested in closing the case. As Coroner, I had no jurisdiction. Wearing my "citizen hat," however, I felt a major public hazard existed which needed to be addressed sooner rather than later.

My email to the Director of the Environmental Protection Agency in Washington, D.C., copied to the Idaho Congressional delegation, resulted in a call from the local EPA office in Coeur d'Alene informing me they were taking emergency intervention in the case.

The next day, there were several suburban vans with tinted windows and a crew of EPA agents at the Church Road location. They confiscated approximately 18,000 6-oz. canisters of propane/butane (HC12). Approximately, one third of the canisters were rusted or leaking. They removed the two bulk tanks of propane and butane from the property as well.

The Oz Technologies web site remains active. I do not know if any of the canisters reached retailers or were ever installed as a refrigerant in vehicles. I fault several local and federal agencies for not intervening before this accident. The bulk propane/butane gas suppliers must have been aware of the business practices ongoing at the site. No legal action resulted from the case.

Fire Investigators learned that Lindgren would fill the canisters in his mobile home under unsafe conditions. An ignition source from either the water heater or the washer/dryer probably set off the explosion and fire.

I learned that if you push the right buttons, even the EPA will respond quickly and appropriately.

Incidentally, Lindgren has been lionized in several alternative publications and Web sites as a visionary persecuted by DuPont, Inc. (the owners of the HFC patents) and the federal government.

*     *     *

## Radon

Radon (atomic weight (AW) 222 and 226) is a radioactive, colorless, odorless gas emitted by the degradation of Uranium (AW 238). The various rocks and soils, deposited in North Idaho by the massive Lake Missoula floods, derive from erosion of the Rocky Mountains. Radioactive uranium is one of the components of these rocks.

*Radon levels in houses (as well as schools and other buildings) have registered radon levels at four to forty times the acceptable level for human exposure. The EPA has recommended remediation for buildings with greater than 4.0 picocuries/liter of air. Since 1970, contractors have installed impermeable plastic membranes beneath foundations and walls. Testing kits and/or commercial contractors are used to measure radon levels. Home remediation measures chiefly address ventilation of crawl spaces or installing negative pressure systems to gather the radon gas from beneath the foundation and vent it to outside air. Oncologists believe that radon is responsible for more than 80% of the lung cancer in non-smokers.*

*A delightful forty-five-year-old CPA was found to have metastatic small-cell lung cancer. A life long non-smoker, her home had a radon level of 18 picocuries/liter of air. Her oncologist diagnosed her tumor as etiologically due to radon exposure. The long interval between radiation exposure and the development of the cancers make this a difficult problem for coroners to diagnose and catalogue for Vital Statistics. However, when the evidence indicates a strong relationship to the cause of death, it should be included for the record.*

*Another radiation issue relates to the wartime $I^{131}$ releases from plutonium production at the Hanford Site in Central Washington during the so-called "Green run." Eastern Washington and North Idaho are "downwind" from the site. The radioactive elements rained down on grass, which was in-turn ingested by dairy cows and expressed in their milk. Humans, especially infants, who ingested the milk, had the iodine isotope concentrated in the thyroid gland. Several cases of hypothyroidism, thyroid cancer and other cancers were attributed to the Hanford release.*

The "Downwinders," as they were called, only partially prevailed in their protracted lawsuit against the federal government contractors, E.I. DuPont and General Electric. Settlements as low as $25,000 were offered and accepted by some victims with hypothyroidism and/or thyroid cancer.[10] The lawsuit brought attention to preventative measures in the event that such radiation occurs in the future.

Note: The 2011 earthquake and tsunami resulted in radiation leaks from the damaged the nuclear reactors at Fukoshima, Japan. Health authorities made widespread recommendations for using Potassium Iodide tablets to block the thyroid from concentrating iodine in the gland.

---

[10] "Settlements Being Readied for Some Downwinders" Environmental Defense Institute, Vol. 21, Number 8, December 2010.

# CHAPTER 13

# "DUMPSTER DIVING FOR DUMMIES"

Garbage and recyclables are collected in dumpsters placed around the county at various collection sites, as well as curbside barrels. Waste Management Corp. has the contract for collecting the garbage, which is hauled to two transfer stations and later delivered to the county landfill. The recyclable material is taken to a sorting facility where contents are sorted and shipped to various commercial recycling plants.

*I was called to examine two human skulls found in a rural county garbage dumpster. We were able to track down the source from other materials collected from the dumpster. The individual admitted to disposing of the skulls, which had been in his possession for several years. The possession of a skull is not illegal. However, how it was obtained is another matter. In addition, we are very conscious of the traditions and practices of the Coeur d'Alene tribe in regards to such matters.*

*The individual stated that his aunt and uncle gave him the skulls which they had collected during travels to Southeast Asia and New Guinea. He moved to Coeur d'Alene several years ago and kept the skulls in a box in his garage. He decided to discard them while cleaning his garage. There was no way we could confirm or deny his story. It was important to establish that these were not of Native American origin. I consulted with a forensic anthropologist at Eastern Washington University, who agreed to examine* the skulls using an anthropomorphic parameter computer program available through her professional contacts.

Using a series of skull measurements including facial characteristics, inter-orbital distances and other parameters, she was able to ascertain that the skulls were consistent with Southeast Asian origin and did not conform to parameters associated with Native North Americans. We thus avoided what might have been an unpleasant confrontation with tribal members whose reverence for their ancestors and burial traditions would have presented problems for the authorities.

Another instance was not as pleasant. A dumpster designated for cardboard recyclables was located at Lakes Middle School in Coeur d'Alene. In October, a homeless person was sleeping under cardboard cartons in the dumpster. A Waste Management truck driver inserted the truck's lift forks into the side lifting brackets, hoisted the dumpster, and dumped the contents into the truck hopper. Hydraulic rams compressed the contents.

The truck proceeded to other pickup locations and eventually returned to the sorting facility where workers found the compressed body of the transient. We were able to make identification from papers found on the body but it was a traumatic experience for the personnel, as well as for the "dumpster diver."

On another occasion, one January evening, I responded to a residence in Coeur d'Alene at the request of the Coeur d'Alene police. On a "welfare check" they found an elderly female's body wrapped in a rug in the back of a Volkswagen van. Because of the below-freezing conditions, there were little signs of decomposition. Her son, who lived with her in the residence, was "intellectually challenged."

Under further questioning, he related his mother stated previously that when she died she wanted to return to her native South Dakota. After her death at home, he wrapped her in the rug, placed her in his van and drove to South Dakota. When he got there, he drove to a remote road but could not bring himself to dump the body in a snow bank. He turned around and drove back to Coeur d'Alene and parked the van at his house. Neighbors became concerned and called the police.

A local funeral home transported the body. She was buried in a Coeur d'Alene cemetery. The cause and manner of death was determined to be of natural causes. The County Prosecutor decided not to prosecute the son for unlawful body transport across state lines. He felt that due to the son's mental status, he was unable to comprehend the consequences of his decision to transport the body to South Dakota and back.

## CHAPTER 14

# DOMESTIC VIOLENCE AND HOMICIDE

It is not possible to estimate the incidence of domestic violence in Kootenai County, or nationally. The majority of cases never come to the attention of the coroner. Emergency-room physicians document numerous cases each year, while charges are seldom pursued due to the victim's unwillingness to press charges, or fear of retribution. A discussion of the various etiologic reasons, or causes, involved in domestic abuse cases goes far beyond the scope of this book. The coroner relies on the "eyes and ears" of law enforcement, first responders, KMC emergency department personnel and morticians, to help in identifying which of these cases warrant further investigation.

*Sheriff Pierce Clegg called me one frigid January 2 night to a home in a gated subdivision in the Meadowbrook area south of Coeur d'Alene. Ambient temperatures were near zero.*

*A retired anesthesiologist and his wife moved from California to the Coeur d'Alene area. Out-of-state family members became concerned about the whereabouts of the wife. When they asked the physician where she was, he gave vague answers about her going to visit a relative locally. On another occasion, he stated she had gone to California to visit children. KCSO investigated further and obtained a search warrant. The frozen body of the wife was discovered in the garage. Deputies secured the scene and took the doctor into custody.*

*Investigating deputies escorted me through the house. The main level of the house was decorated in a Southwestern motif with many Mexican tiles and art objects. The interior was immaculate and spotless. I would characterize the house as almost "sterile." When we went to the lower level, however, there was a decided odor of decomposition. The murderer had wrapped the body in a throw-rug and stashed it behind a water heater. After several days, body fluids began leaking from the body. Bloody drag patterns from the water heater led to a ground-level entry and a walkway leading to the garage.*

*An autopsy confirmed the woman had been strangled, and showed other signs of abuse. The physician was charged with the murder. The problem was, when taken into custody, he showed signs of severe dementia. He was of little help in notifying family members in California. Physicians who examined him found him to be suffering from Alzheimer's disease. He was institutionalized and later died. We retained her mandible for dental identification in the event that any questions arose after the body was transported back to California for burial. Fortunately, there were no problems, and this tragic case was closed.*

Police and Law Enforcement members occasionally have to deal with distraught family members and other bystanders when investigating crime scenes.

*Coeur d'Alene Police escorted me through a raucous crowd of bystanders and inebriated family members into a home where the husband had fired a rifle at his wife, which resulted in a massive head wound. The blast scattered blood and brain matter along a hallway and into the bedroom. Officers removed a domestic cat which was disturbing crime scene elements. I completed my investigation and had the funeral home transport the body to the SCME for autopsy.*

Once again, the circumstances of the event, documentation of various skeletal fragments and blood spatter patterns, and estimating the distance from the weapon to the victim, are a joint effort with the police investigator. When the case comes to trial, the coroner and police detective plus the forensic pathologist will be called upon to present the results of their investigations.

One of the mysteries of North Idaho is: "Why do the most bizarre cases occur in the midst of the worst possible weather?"

*I responded to a crime scene near Twin Lakes after a series of blizzards blocked roads and limited visibility. KCSO deputies responded to a residence after the son received a phone call from his father saying there had been an altercation and he had killed his wife.*

*When the deputies arrived at the home, the father barricaded himself in the home. They heard a single gunshot, entered the home, and found the victim with a gunshot wound (GSW) to the head. He was transported to Kootenai Medical Center with non-life threatening injuries.*

*Heavy-duty snow removal equipment sat in the yard: a bulldozer, grader, and large front-end loader, which had piled snow in fifteen-foot-high berms to clear a parking area. Huge piles of snow ringed the farmyard, with twelve-foot banks of snow lining the driveway. I parked my vehicle several hundred yards down the access road behind one of the sheriff vehicles.*

*We found his wife's body under some carpet in the back of a pickup truck. She had been bludgeoned to death with a trenching tool called a Pulaski. (This tool was created by and named after a famous Silver Valley miner and firefighter, Ed Pulaski)[11]*

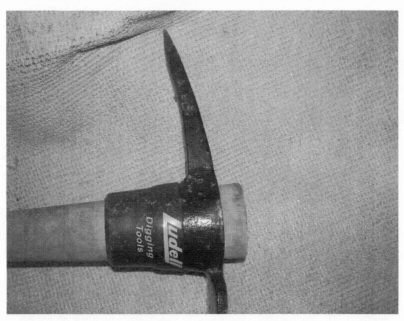

"Pulaski Trenching Tool"

[11]  Kershner, Jim, "Pulaski's Legacy Alive in Standard Fire Tool," Spokesman-Review, August 17, 2010

*Her autopsy listed the cause of death as multiple blunt-force traumatic injuries. The husband survived his self-inflicted GSW, and was convicted of homicide and sentenced to prison.*

Other cases are more subtle, and rely on careful history-taking by emergency department personnel, first responders, and physicians. When the history of a fall downstairs does not conform to usual circumstances, it raises the question of whether the fall was accidental, or from other causes. Head or cervical spine injuries from such falls may be accompanied by other signs of abuse, such as healed fractures or bruising.

The history given by the patient may differ from that of the spouse or other family members. An index of suspicion can be crucial in determining whether cases are the result of abuse. Most of these cases do not fall under the jurisdiction of the Coroner's Office. When the victim succumbs after surgery or several days in the intensive care unit, it may be difficult or impossible to backtrack and get the real story.

The death certificate is routed to the Coroner's Office whenever there are accidental injuries listed as the cause of death. We spend considerable time revising death certificates which may have listed a death as "natural," and list the sequence of events leading to death. For example: "Pneumonia due to: post-op evacuation of subdural hematoma, due to: fall, down staircase."

Dexter Yates, a local funeral director and I have presented several in-service sessions to the Kootenai Medical Center staff in an effort to clarify the process of death certificate completion.

*One of my breast cancer patients came to my office for follow-up. Although her breast exam was normal, I noted multiple chest bruises and several fractured ribs. After additional questioning, she told me her husband had beaten her several days previously and thrown her down a flight of stairs. Nonetheless, she planned to return to her husband.*

*I called the husband into the exam room, explained my concerns, and advised him to get anger management counseling. I further advised him that if she succumbed or died under suspicious circumstances, there would be a careful investigation for cause and manner of death with him as a person of interest. Thankfully, she did not appear with more injuries.*

# CHAPTER 15

# SUDDEN UNEXPECTED INFANT DEATHS (SUID) (INCLUDING SIDS)

No parent is prepared for the discovery of a limp, cyanotic, non-breathing infant. Despite prompt resuscitative measures, these infants often die. The coroner must conduct a careful, compassionate and prompt death investigation in all such cases. This is difficult under the circumstances when the parents are grieving, and frequently resist such investigations.

The American Academy of Pediatrics (AAP) issued guidelines for the prevention of SIDS in 1992. These resulted in a 55% decrease in SIDS deaths by 20011.

First, a definition of SIDS: "The sudden death of a post-neonatal infant under the age of one whose death remains unknown after full investigation including autopsy and toxicology." [Source: American Academy of Pediatrics (AAP) and the *Centers of Disease Control Bulletin*.] The recommendations include:

- Non-prone sleeping position
- Firm sleeping surface
- Avoid soft bedding
- Avoid overheating
- Avoid exposure to tobacco smoke or alcohol

- Routine immunizations
- Bed sharing vs. room sharing
- Maternal use of prescription or non-prescription drugs or alcohol, which may result in toxic levels in breast milk.

More recently, the term Sudden Unexpected Infant Death (SUID) has been utilized to better categorize these tragic deaths. A SUID Case Registry, funded by the National Center for Child Death Review, has subdivided the causes of infant deaths. SIDS still accounts for 50% of such deaths. Accidental suffocation, cardiac arrhythmias, inborn errors of metabolism, infections and poisoning or overdose plus a small residual group of cases listed as "unknown" comprise the remainder.

The coroner must ensure a careful, compassionate and thorough investigation of both the accident scene, and interview of parents or caregivers. This includes salient facts such as:

- Temperature of the location where the baby was found
- If the crib has drop-rail sides (now illegal)
- The presence of extra-soft pillows or bedding
- If the baby was sleeping on a sofa or on a bed where he/she might slip between the mattress or cushions, or the wall or headboard.

Other questions may bring a reasonable cause to light. Researchers have found it helpful to use a baby manikin for the parent or caregiver to use to "walk" through the incident.

While all this may seem intrusive for grieving parents, it is necessary to gain an understanding of the causes of SUID. It also is helpful for those who may counsel parents of possible problems in subsequent pregnancies. There is a slightly increased association of SUID when a prior sibling has died of SIDS/SUID. The bottom line: it is not sufficient to label an infant death as "SIDS" unless a full investigation has been carried out. It is our protocol, and the recommendation of the American Academy of Pediatrics, to autopsy all SUID cases, with the exception of previously known conditions incompatible with life.

The issue of maternal smothering while nursing or bed sharing is actually quite rare. If there has been maternal substance abuse, notably alcohol or illicit drugs—which dull the awareness and senses—the rates go up. These are all items, which must be considered in investigating such cases.

"Shaken Baby Syndrome" is particularly troubling, and may come to light in the emergency room when an infant is brought in with head injuries, or retinal bleeding. Parents, as well as "significant others" or babysitters, are often the perpetrators.

Conflicting stories or gaps in the timeline are some of the warning flags when abuse may have occurred. It is important for interviews to be conducted individually, rather than conference style. The skills of the interviewer are critical to getting a cogent and complete history.

Admittedly, the coroner or the police investigator may not be the best person to do the interviews. They need to be conducted by a person experienced in interview techniques to obtain accurate information and, at the same time, cause the least distress to grieving family members.

# CHAPTER 16

# TREES, LOGS
# AND LOGGERS

The timber industry is central to understanding the history and development of Idaho. Timber harvest in the millions of board feet of lumber from the Panhandle National Forest and other private lands supply the mills in Kootenai County. The last of the log drives down the Clearwater River was in 1971. Loggers piled huge decks of saw logs on the banks of the river edge until the spring runoff began. They released the decks and the logs crashed into the river to begin the ninety-mile journey down the Clearwater River to the Potlatch Lumber mill at Lewiston, Idaho. Lumberjacks in jet-drive workboats would clamber onto logjams with pike poles, peaveys and, occasionally, explosive charges to break up the jams and get the masses of logs moving again.

It was very dangerous work. H. Don Moseley, M.D., a Coeur d'Alene physician, accompanied the last Clearwater log drive, riding on the "Wanigan" floating cookhouse and bunkhouse. That unique experience will never be repeated in North Idaho.

Logging remains in the top ten most hazardous occupations in this country. Some of the reasons behind the hazards of this job involve steep terrain, foul weather, unstable or diseased trees and certain time/work constraints.

Watching a logger at work is a thing of beauty. Selecting a tree for felling, he makes an undercut on the "down" side and proceeds to finish the cut with his chainsaw, using wedges to ensure that the tree falls in the predetermined direction. Once down, the logger limbs the branches and cuts it into sixteen and a half-foot sections, then skidded to the loading site.

Unfortunately, it does not always happen this smoothly. The top third of a hundred-foot pine may snap off without warning and strike the logger, or others on the ground. The tree may "hang up" in surrounding trees—the infamous "widow maker"—which is even more dangerous.

In 1989, my good friend and experienced logger, Richard White contracted to log a portion of our family's lake property which had fifty years of neglected forest and a nearly impenetrable tangle of deadfalls and downed trees piled like giant pick-up sticks. We aimed to log the marketable timber and pile the slash in burn piles. He methodically worked upslope, carefully selecting the sound trees, scaling the logs and skidded them down to Coeur d'Alene Lake. I watched from a safe distance as the trees were felled, limbed and cut to size. In all, we had 55,000 board feet of logs impounded at our docks. The log barge from one of the mills came and loaded the logs for transport to the mill. We had twenty-four slash piles, each as big as a small house. It took six weeks of steady fire-tending to finally consume the burn piles. Richard would *not* allow this amateur to use his chainsaw, but he would let "Doc" pile and burn slash until the summer burn-ban season. The net result has been an open forest with new growth trees, abundant wildlife and hiking trails that we all enjoy. In addition, elimination of the huge fuel source has reduced the seasonal fire danger.

Other loggers, and would-be loggers, were not so fortunate. I made multiple coroner calls in the Panhandle National Forest to investigate logging accidents.

*A contract logging crew comprised of Guatemalan guest workers had a Douglas fir snap off its top third and strike another logger who was working below the crew. The crew spoke only Spanish and it took several hours to sound the alarm and for KCSO to respond to the Carlin Bay road site. It took another hour for the Coroner to drive around the lake and find his way to the parked sheriff vehicle, clamber down to examine the body and the smashed safety helmet, get copies of the passport and identification, then get the funeral home transport personnel on scene for removal. A formal industrial investigation determined that the manner of death was accidental. Making notification to next of kin was likewise encumbered by the communication with relatives in Guatemala to arrange transport of the body home.*

Most people who live in the Northwest are accustomed to seeing huge log loads on the highways. The logs are loaded by cranes or self-loading hydraulic booms and secured by multiple binder cables drawn tightly over the load.

*One 53 year-old logging truck driver was securing his load at the work site. The foreman found him deceased alongside his truck. The assumption was that he experienced a cardiac event as the cause of death. Because it no one witnessed his death, and due to the industrial nature of the case, we sent the body for autopsy. Surprisingly, very little coronary artery disease was present. The forensic pathologist noted changes in the micro sections of the heart muscle consistent with electrocution.*

*The body had been released to the funeral home. I went there to make an additional examination. I saw multiple exit burns on the feet and toes corresponding to the caulk nails on his logging boots. Sections taken from the foot burns confirmed the electrical nature of the burns.*

*The mystery was solved when we investigated the job site. The trucker had tossed the binder cable over the load and across an adjacent power line, which electrocuted him. Again, careful observation at the scene and at the medical examiner's facility was a key factor in determining the accidental, rather than natural, cause of death.*

\* \* \*

*The Forest Service issues firewood permits to private individuals who use wood stoves for home heating.*

*A Kellogg logger was working in the Killarney Peak area when he sustained massive head injuries from a 'widow-maker.' Responding, I drove east on Interstate 90 to the Fourth of July Pass and followed USFS Rd. 614 to a communications relay site at Killarney Peak. A USFS law enforcement official then directed me to the accident scene a hundred yards downslope.*

*As I descended the hillside, I noted several similar widow-makers. I used extreme caution as I approached the scene where Detective Maskell waited. There were two chainsaws at the site, one belonging to the victim and another from another logger in the party.*

*Once we completed our investigation, we discussed whether Central Dispatch had alerted the funeral home personnel to come to the scene. With approaching darkness and a weather forecast of an imminent snowstorm, I decided to initiate transport up the slope to my SUV. Detective Maskell and another deputy claimed back problems so the USFS enforcement official and I hauled the body up to my SUV, where we placed the victim in a second body bag. When I was finally able to establish cell phone coverage at the I-90 on-ramp at Fourth of July Summit, funeral home personnel indicated they were just leaving their parking lot. I cancelled their transport and delivered the body to the funeral home.*

Although, "just part of the job," my back was sore for several days thereafter. I reminded the funeral home personnel they owed me a Starbucks Latte for the transport.

The National Forests are a latticework of designated USFS roads and numerous non-designated trails remaining from previous logging sites. In addition, snow comes early and stays late in the woods. Too many I-90 drivers leave the freeway to explore Forest Service Roads and/or logging roads, only to get stuck in a snow bank or run off the road. Cell phone coverage is limited and, without a trip plan in place, the situation can rapidly become critical. As temperatures plummet, either their fuel is exhausted or the car battery runs down. They are seldom equipped to survive the elements. Occasionally, a snowmobiler will come upon the vehicle and notify Back Country Rescue teams to effect a recovery. It is my practice to wait for their transport to Coeur d'Alene rather than run the risk of becoming a casualty myself.

Infrequently, as hypothermia sets in, individuals begin shedding their clothes in a false perception that they are over-heating.

*We found two males nearly nude near Rose Lake in January. They had abandoned their disabled car and tried to hike out for help. We found a trail of clothing, coats, etc. along their footprints in the snow as they moved away from their car.*

Lumber mills are another work location wherein hazards are an ever-present danger.

*One worker was sorting planks as they came off a trim- saw machine. A six-foot long trim section caught on the chain "dog" and was propelled into his abdomen at high speed. He was initially taken to the Sandpoint hospital where the 'missile' was removed prior to his transfer to Kootenai Medical Center. We stabilized his condition, started broad-spectrum antibiotics, and gave him a tetanus shot before taking him to surgery. The wooden spear tracked through several loops of small intestine, into the pancreas and alongside the common bile duct, inferior vena cava and into the posterior abdominal muscles. He eventually recovered after a series of secondary procedures to re-establish intestinal continuity. He was extremely fortunate that removal of the foreign body had not resulted in a fatal hemorrhage.*

In the mills, wood scraps are fed by conveyors to boilers, which produce power for the mill, and steam to dry and cure the finished lumber.

*A worker doing maintenance on the conveyor became entrapped in the mechanism and was fatally injured. I went to the plywood mill to assess the accident scene, and to produce a death investigation report for the Idaho industrial commission. They, in turn, developed safety recommendations to prevent a recurrence of such injuries.*

# CHAPTER 17

# HOMICIDE IN KOOTENAI COUNTY AND IDAHO

Homicide is an uncommon crime in Idaho. The homicide rate in Idaho from 1960–2010 ranged from 1.8 to 3.3 per 100,000 residents. This range of variability reflects Idaho's population growth from 690,000 in 1960 to more than 1.6 million people in 2012. The U.S homicide rate is 4.7 per 100,000 based on the most recent available data (CDC 2010). International statistics are not exactly comparable because of reporting differences and other factors. When a homicide does occur, Idaho coroners and law enforcement members face all of the factors which agencies in Los Angeles or New York encounter on a more regular basis. Those agencies, however, work many more cases per year and possess the resources to deal with them. Idaho Death Investigators, both law enforcement and coroners, may be relatively inexperienced in the issues involved in homicide investigation.

*June 17, 1998, was a dark day in Idaho Law Enforcement history. Linda Huff, 33, an Idaho State Police officer, became the first ISP officer slain in the line of duty. At 11 p.m. on that date, she was reporting for duty at the ISP regional office. Scott D. Yager, 33, accosted her in the parking lot and shot her seventeen times—the last shot an execution-type contact wound to the head. Though gravely injured, Officer Huff was able to empty her .45-caliber Smith & Wesson service revolver striking Yager in the shoulder and mouth.*

*Idaho State Police and multiple regional law enforcement personnel responded in force, apprehending Yager as he walked away from the scene.*

*When I arrived at the chaotic scene, the deceased ten-year veteran of law enforcement lay on the parking lot pavement covered with a blood-soaked sheet. Her bullet-proof vest had withstood several bullet impacts. She suffered multiple other wounds, one of which severed her spinal cord. She was pronounced dead at the scene.*

*It is difficult to describe the level of hostility and anger present among the responding law enforcement officers when "one of their own" is gunned down. Medical personnel had already transported Yager to Kootenai Medical Center for treatment of his non-life threatening wounds. He was hospitalized under armed guard.*

*The Kootenai County Sheriff's Office assumed the investigation. In Officer-involved shootings, it is customary to have another law enforcement agency handle the investigation to maintain an impartial, thorough investigation without the influence of emotions which might cloud professional performance and to prevent any suggestion of cover-up.*

*Likewise, I found myself with conflicting emotions as I examined the fallen officer: the mother of three and the wife of another ISP officer. As with all such cases, however, my duty was to the deceased. I knew that when Yager's inevitable trial was conducted, defense attorneys would argue against the prosecution's case.*

*The autopsy was conducted by the Spokane Medical Examiner (SCME) to document the heinous nature of her injuries and to buttress the argument that this case was one of "aggravated murder of a police officer," which would allow prosecutors to ask for the death penalty. Yager had ridden his bicycle to the scene and committed the premeditated crime without any extenuating circumstances.*

*At trial, the District Court judge would not allow the "aggravated murder of a police officer" charge. Scott Yager was convicted and sentenced to life in prison without chance of parole on August 19, 1999.*

In 2005, Linda Huff was posthumously awarded the first Idaho Law Enforcement and Firefighter Medal of Honor. Her name adorns the Regional ISP Crime Laboratory in Coeur d'Alene.

Her death illustrates the requirement for constant vigilance on the part of law enforcement to ensure their safety and protection, even as they stand in the line of duty each and every day. It also illustrates how coroners must understand their responsibility to investigate crimes without regard to personal feelings of anger, fear or revenge. The documentation of the facts is critical to put each piece of the puzzle in place so prosecutors and juries clearly understand the case as they deliberate.

## Murder, Intrigue and Cunning Deception

The following complex case remains a puzzle in many ways. We have four people dead, another in prison, a missing child (now 23, if alive) and more questions than answers for all of the agencies involved.

*November 13, 1995: A KCSO patrol officer called me to a homicide scene on Seely Road off Seltice Way. A nearby resident heard a gunshot about 3:30 A.M., but saw no disturbance outside. He later observed a newspaper carrier's Toyota Camry stationary at the delivery boxes with its lights on. He investigated, found the body and called authorities.*

*The driver, later identified as **Gary C. Loesch, age 55,** was slumped over to the right with a large bloodstain on the upholstery. There were several November 13 issues of the Spokesman-Review wrapped in waterproof sleeves. Additional bound bundles lay in the back seat. A single gunshot wound was noted in the left malar area, with no apparent exit wound.*

*Two filtered cigarette butts were at the base of a large ponderosa pine nearest the delivery boxes. A single set of tire tracks led up Seely Road to the intersection with Seltice Way. KCSO deputies secured the scene and began a search of the area for additional evidence. The victim's son, **Charles Loesch,** arrived at the scene and was interviewed by officers. He had attempted to locate his father when he failed to return from his paper route. The last reported sighting was at 2:30 A.M. when the victim and his brother received their shipments of the morning papers.*

*The victim's hands were secured with paper bags for later barium testing for gunpowder residue. Following KCSO's completion of their scene investigation, the body was removed and taken to SCME for autopsy.*

*The Forensic Institute autopsy report showed:*

I.  Shotgun wound to the head:
    A.  Site of entrance: left cheek
    B.  Site of exit: none
    C.  Direction of fire: left to right, anterior to posterior and slightly upward
    D:  Track of missile: through left cheek, posterior oropharynx, entering cranial cavity through base of middle cranial fossa and through the midbrain and cerebellum with extensive tissue pulpefaction
    E.  Associated injuries: cerebral pulpefaction, subarachnoid hemorrhage, aspiration of blood into tracheobronchial airways; cranial vault and basal skull fractures
    F.  Missile recovery: pellet samples from cranial tissues, including components of wadding.
II. Atherosclerotic cardiovascular disease
III. Mild exogenous obesity

We classified the manner of death as homicide. The murder weapon was never found, although Post Falls Police did recover a shotgun from a closet in the victim's home. The bluing on the gun had been removed with some type of abrasive material. I am not aware of the gauge, make or model of the gun. The case remained an open investigation.

***January 11, 1998:*** *Post Falls Police discovered a body, later identified as **Barbara D. Loesch (age 54,)** floating in a hot tub on the back deck of her home. A TV was found in the hot tub. A long extension cord connected to the TV was disconnected at the wall outlet in the garage. My Chief Deputy Coroner, Jody DeLuca Hissong responded to the scene. She ordered the body taken to the SCME for autopsy. The victim's daughter, **Tina Loesch**, was interviewed and stated she last saw Barbara alive on January 8, 1998.*

*The autopsy report listed:*

I. Scene and Circumstances compatible with potential asphyxia by drowning with:
    A. No definite evidence of traumatic injury
    B. No intrinsic disease state sufficient to have caused death
II. Moderate putrefactive changes compatible with substantial interval of time in warm hot tub
III. Status post cholecystectomy and appendectomy
IV. Minimal aortic atherosclerosis

*"Opinion: This decedent was found expired in a hot tub. Judging from the last time she was known alive, and other circumstantial information, it appears she may have expired on approximately January 8, 1998, with the body remaining in the hot tub thereafter. At autopsy no traumatic injury could definitely be identified. No natural disease state sufficient to have caused death was identified."*

*Due to multiple uncertain facts in the case, Deputy Coroner Deluca-Hissong submitted the death certificate to the Idaho Department of Vital Statistics with the following information:*

Item #3:     Date of Death: Between January 8 and January 11, 1998
Item #26:    Manner of Death: Could Not Be Determined
Item #30 a:  Date of Injury: Unknown
Item #30 b:  Hour of Injury: Unknown
Item #30 c:  Description how Injury Occurred: Victim found floating face-down in her hot tub.

***Tina Loesch**, daughter of the decedent, was interviewed by Post Falls Police who found insufficient evidence to charge her with any crime. The Post Falls Police treated the case as an accident, but had many concerns about the case.*

*Tina Loesch had been incarcerated in the women's prison in Boise for a number of years. While she was in prison, her son, **Kristopher C. Loesch**, age sixteen, was cared for by Barbara Loesch. He later moved to the Spokane*

*Valley, Washington to live with **Steven Cassell**. Cassell is married to **Julie Twyford**, the attorney for Tina Loesch.*

*While in prison, Tina began a relationship with another inmate, **Skye Hanson**. The two women returned to Kootenai County after their release from prison. The women set up a home remodel/renovation business in Pullman, WA, where they lived.*

*One of their remodel jobs was for an elderly widow named **Dorothy Martin**. Mrs. Martin usually wore a large diamond ring which she often displayed to visitors. Tina and Skye had one of their employees, **Bradley Steckman**, break into the Martin home, intent on stealing the ring. Unfortunately, Mrs. Martin awoke during the robbery. Steckman smothered her with a pillow and escaped with the ring. Pullman police later arrested and charged him with murder. He was convicted and sentenced to a western Washington correctional unit.*

*In 2003, Steckman contacted authorities and admitted his part in the plot to murder both Gary and Barbara Loesch. Bradley Steckman was aware that Tina Loesch became very angry when she discovered her father, Gary Loesch, had rewritten his will as a consequence of her lesbian relationship with Skye Hanson. According to Fred Gabourie, a retired Coeur d'Alene attorney who rewrote the will, Gary left Tina one dollar, while the remainder of his estate was to go to her brother, **Charles Loesch**. Steckman denied shooting Gary Loesch but did admit that he had scoped out his newspaper route.*

*Steckman related the following scenario to Post Falls Police in 2003:*

*Tina had gradually resumed a normal mother/daughter relationship with her mother, thanking her for the care of her son while she was in prison, and generally appearing to care for her well-being. Tina, Skye and Bradley Steckman were visitors at the Post Falls home and the home-remodeling business they were involved with seemed to thrive. Tina also purchased a $500,000 life insurance policy on Barbara's life from Midland Insurance Company with herself as the beneficiary. The policy matured in 1988, prior to Barbara's death.*

*Tina bought her mother a small TV, which she placed on the deck to watch while relaxing in the jetted hot tub. An extension cord from a receptacle in the garage powered the TV. On January 8, 1998, the trio shared dinner and drinks with Barbara Loesch. Barbara was bothered with chronic back pain and readily agreed to Tina's suggestion that they all get in the hot tub, have some drinks, and enjoy the TV.*

*The trio had previously hatched a plan to murder Barbara. After an interval in the tub, Steckman got out getting another beer, Tina and Skye also got out, on some pretense, leaving Barbara alone in the hot tub. Bradley Steckman returned with his beer and "pretended" to stumble, knocking the TV into the hot tub. The high voltage transformer in the TV shocked, but did not kill, Barbara. Steckman unplugged the extension cord at the outlet. Tina Loesch then forcibly held Barbara's head underwater until she drowned. The trio then removed all evidence of their presence in the home and left the scene. Barbara Loesch's body was found three days later.*

*Tina Loesch and Bradley Steckman were questioned and released by Post Falls Police. The police initially treated the case as an accident. Tina Loesch proceeded to have her attorney, Julie Twyford, pressure the Coroner's Office to issue a death certificate, so she could submit a claim for the $500,000 death benefit on her mother's life insurance. Midland Insurance Company paid the claim based on the death certificate we had filed, listing the cause and manner of death as "could not be determined" as detailed above.*

*Once they received the check and deposited it in Skye Hanson's bank account, the couple disappeared, as did Kristopher Loesch on or about May 16, 2001.*

*Based on Steckman's confession, murder warrants were issued for Tina Loesch and Skye Hanson. Steckman was charged with lesser charges and returned to the Washington prison system to serve his sentence concurrently with his sentence in the Dorothy Martin murder.*

*On September 29, 2003, we filed an affidavit with Idaho Vital Statistics Department correcting the date of death to January 8, 1988, with the cause of death: "fresh-water drowning due to forced manual submersion and electric shock." The manner of death was changed to: "Homicide."*

*NOTE: This is illustrative of why we submit death certificates as either "Pending" or "Cannot be Determined" If, as in this case, new information is obtained, the cause and manner can be changed once, but only one time.*

*A nationwide search for the fugitives produced few clues. The case went cold for five years. Kristopher Loesch—a.k.a. Kristopher (Christopher)*

*Robinson or Robin Loesch, or Robin Kessler—was placed on the Missing and Exploited Children list.*

*In November 2008, the case was profiled on the national TV documentary "America's Most Wanted." Within hours of the airing of the program, the bodies of Tina Loesch, age 37 and Skye Hanson, age 44, were found in their Dodge Durango outside of Tucson, Arizona. They died from gunshot wounds to the head in an apparent murder/suicide pact.*

*The Pima County (AZ) Medical Examiner determined that Tina shot Skye in the head and then turned the weapon on herself. Both died instantly. A six-page suicide note was found with the bodies. The note did not take the blame for either parent's death.*

*Kristopher Loesch remains missing. He would be twenty-three years old (as of November 2013). He apparently lived with Tina (a.k.a. "Dawn") and Skye (a.k.a. "Katie") in about 2002. Tina told her neighbors she had sent Kristopher to Seattle to live with relatives there. There is no confirmation of that information.*

Any information regarding the case of Kristopher Loesch would be of great help in finally resolving this case. The contact number for the National Center for Missing and Exploited Children is 1-800-843-5678.

# CHAPTER 18

# JOSEPH E. DUNCAN, III AND THE GROENE-MACKENSIE MURDERS

*May 2005:* The red Jeep Cherokee with Missouri license plates stopped on the shoulder of the westbound lane of Interstate 90 in the Wolf Lodge area east of Coeur d'Alene did not attract much attention. The driver, **Joseph E. Duncan, III, age 44**, had spent nearly half his life in prison for sexual assault, parole violations and other crimes.

The convicted felon spent several minutes scanning a nearby home where two children, **Shasta (age8) and Dylan Groene (age9)**, ran through a lawn sprinkler in the yard. A Coeur d'Alene school bus stopped and **Slade Groene (age 13)** got off the bus and entered the house. Later, Slade crossed the meadow to mow the lawn for a neighbor, **Robert "Bob" Hollingsworth**. Slade later returned home. An adult male, **Mark Mackenzie age 37,** returned from work, parked his pickup in the driveway and entered the house.

After several minutes, the Jeep Cherokee then merged with traffic and proceeded on I-90 to Spokane, Washington. Once there, Duncan posed as a rental prospect and toured two apartments. The next evening, and for several days thereafter, Duncan drove the Jeep back to the Wolf Lodge area. He scanned the area with binoculars and night-vision goggles, noting the comings and goings of Mackenzie, the three children, and their mother, **Brenda Groene, age 40.**

***May 16, 2005:*** *With a light rain falling near sundown, Hollingsworth drove over to the Groene home to pay Slade twenty dollars for mowing his lawn. He also wanted to ask that the white pickup truck, belonging to Dan and Lisa Miller, parked near his home be moved. There was no activity around the home. Hollingsworth knocked on the back door. Hearing no answer, he opened the unlocked door and immediately saw two bodies on the kitchen floor. He backed out of the house and called 911.*

*Kootenai County Sheriff's deputies responded to the scene and secured a perimeter. The responding deputies checked the house, noted three bodies inside and called for investigators. Hollingsworth also told them that Shasta and Dylan Groene were missing.*

*Detective Brad Maskell, Chief Investigator, arrived on scene. By then it was dark, the rain had increased in intensity. Considering the dense overgrown grass surrounding the property alongside Wolf Lodge Creek, Detective Maskell decided to set up a wider crime scene perimeter. He initiated a search for the two missing children, and asked the Idaho State Patrol to issue an Amber Alert.*

Thus began the "Duncan, Groene, Mackensie Case" in Kootenai County, which consumed the community and stretched the resources of many agencies to their limits.

*Detective Maskell notified me of the triple homicide around midnight and that two minor children were missing. After some bureaucratic hurdles, authorities issued an Amber Alert for the two children. The immediate area was searched for the missing children. The wetlands near the Groene home were too dangerous to search in the dark. Due to rainy conditions and safety concerns, Detective Maskell decided to assemble an investigative team at the KCSO command center at five o'clock the next morning.*

*By then, the command center was up and running. Multiple agency representatives—the Sherriff's Department, Office of Emergency Management, Coroner, Coeur d'Alene Police, Idaho State Police, and the FBI—assembled for a briefing before heading out to the Groene residence.*

*There, KCSO officers had set up a shelter within the crime perimeter to protect personnel from the elements.*

The one-story house was of cinder block construction with a corrugated metal roof. A variety of vehicles were parked in the yard in various states of repair. A motorcycle and an RV belonging to the Groene's were inspected by detectives. Hollingsworth reported that he had seen a pickup parked on a road near his house. Several USFS road and trail signs adorned the front of the house.

The front door to the house showed extensive bloody handprints. A single tennis shoe lay on the ground. One rear bedroom window was broken out with curtains waving in the breeze. We noted bloody scuffmarks on the outside wall beneath the window. Detective Maskell escorted Deputy Coroner Lynn Acebedo and me past an apparent "failed" septic tank around to the rear-entry of the house.

We donned biohazard gear, shoe covers, and gloves to enter the kitchen. Unwashed dishes lay in the sink, and an opened can of Dinty-Moore stew sat on the stove. At the base of the kitchen table, the body of Slade Groene, his hands and feet bound with duct tape and zip ties lay with his head against the legs of Brenda Groene, her hands and legs also bound with duct tape and nylon zip ties. Her torso crossed the threshold into the living room. Mark Mackenzie, also bound with zip ties and duct tape, lay next to a coffee table with a broken glass top. All three victims had a strip of duct tape around their necks and a duct tape mouth gag in place. A VCR slipcase for the movie "Taking Lives," starring Angelina Jolie, lay on the coffee table. We found the tape in the VCR player for a large-screen TV. The room was in considerable disarray. A single, live 12-gauge shotgun cartridge lay on the living room floor. A white princess phone sat on a side-table with TV remotes on the couch. The walls contained continuous bloodstains down the hall to two bedrooms. A window in the bedroom remained open. The mattress appeared stained with an unknown reddish, brown material. The washer-dryer in a laundry room and bathroom completed the rooms on the first floor

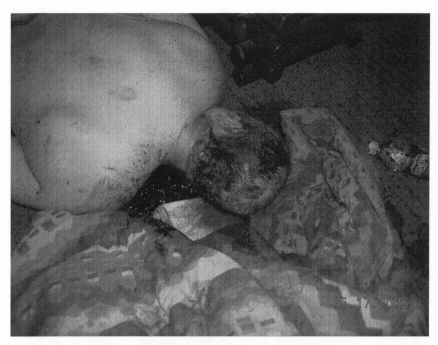

Blunt Head Trauma, Bound Male Victim

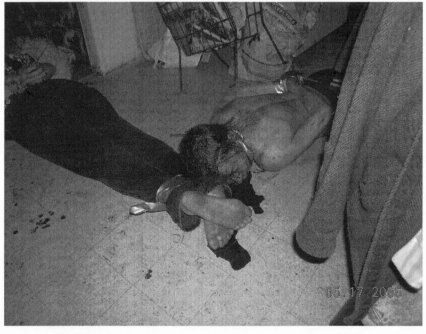

Bound Victims – Groene- Mackensie Homicides

A stairway from the kitchen led up to a sleeping loft, also in disarray. A mattress lay on the floor with its bedding unmade. One dresser contained various articles of female lingerie, blouses and stockings. A second dresser was filled with male underwear and socks.

Returning to the living room, Detective Maskell and the investigating officers were processing the scene. I examined the male victim, identified as Mark Mackenzie, who had been bludgeoned with a blunt instrument. He had several skull fractures with extruded brain material and blood matting his scalp. At least one of the scalp wounds had a clear imprint of a patterned tool-head seen in heavy framing hammers. Brenda and Slade Groene sustained similar head trauma injuries.

Outside, detectives collected evidence from the yard and outbuildings. Detective Maskell insisted that the removal of the bodies be delayed until his investigators obtained all of the evidence needed: DNA, blood and fingerprint samples. The SCME was anxious to have the bodies transported to Spokane for autopsy. I concurred with Detective Maskell that the meticulous processing of all of the evidence obtainable from the scene would take precedence. The exact time of death was of less importance and the cool ambient temperatures would not complicate the autopsy. The multiple injuries the victims sustained were non-survivable. We sent the three bodies for autopsies when KCSO released them from the scene.

In the meantime, an area-wide search was underway for the two missing children. The police interviewed Steve Groene, the father of the children, and his brother. The uncle, with a prior drug-use history, was interviewed and released. We could find no apparent motive for the killing. Various scenarios, such as a drug deal and/or child trafficking abduction were considered. The command center began receiving hundreds of tips and calls around the clock. TV, local and national newspapers ran photos of the missing children.

KCSO Deputies found a white pickup belonging to Dan and Lisa Miller on a side-road near the Hollingsworth residence with rolls of duct tape and 18 inch nylon zip ties in the bed of the truck. (Eventually, Detective Maskell was able to track the Duct Tape to a specific brand only sold in the St. Louis area.)

*Kootenai Search and Rescue on foot, horseback and ATVs made an extensive search of the area. Dive team members searched the deeper pools on Wolf Lodge Creek, as it flowed behind the home and into Coeur d'Alene Lake. Deputies interviewed campers at a nearby campground. Kootenai Jail Work Release inmates sorted through tons of garbage collected from Wolf Lodge dumpsters.*

*As expected, the media frenzy was unprecedented. Satellite trucks, local reporters, and the national networks all descended on Coeur d'Alene within twenty-four hours. One breathless reporter told me that: "Kootenai Search and Rescue had searched '200 acres' on horseback around the home without finding the children." I reminded her that there are one million acres of the Panhandle National Forest adjacent to the Groene home. In addition, another million acres lay in the Lolo National Forest on the Montana side of the border. (Little did I know how that would enter into subsequent events.)Kootenai County Sheriff Rocky Watson delegated Lt. Ben Wolfinger to handle all press releases.*

*Once the Spokane Medical Examiner completed the autopsies, we filed the death certificates with Idaho Vital Statistics. We released the nature of the fatal injuries in general terms. The FBI offered to expedite processing of the DNA and blood samples at their Quantico, Virginia laboratory. An FBI profiler assisted Kootenai authorities in formulating a likely profile of the murderer-kidnapper.*

*During June, the coverage in media subsided, but the missing child posters remained everywhere. Hundreds of tips and clues continued to come into the command center. The KCSO officers continued to process evidence from the scene. School officials had no adverse comments about any of the children. The children's biological father issued pleas for their safe return.*

*On **July 2, 2005,** a man and small girl came into the Denny's Restaurant in Coeur d'Alene about two o'clock in the morning. They ordered a meal from the menu. The girl seemed somewhat withdrawn and disheveled. The waitress recognized the girl from the missing person posters. She went into the kitchen and urgently called 911 for the Coeur d'Alene police to respond to the restaurant for a possible sighting. She then stalled by offering to make the girl a milkshake. Several other denizens of the all-night* restaurant also recognized Shasta and vowed among themselves not to let the girl leave with the as-yet unidentified male. The unidentified male went to the restroom. The waitress asked the girl if she was Shasta Groene, the girl said yes. About that time, the police arrived and arrested Joseph E. Duncan, III without incident.

Shasta was admitted to Kootenai Medical Center, and treated for her multiple injuries. Psychologists interviewed her and began a long process of returning her to a somewhat normal life.

\*    \*    \*

During interviews with Coeur d'Alene police, Shasta told them that her mother called her into the living room where Duncan, wearing gloves, was holding Brenda, Slade and Mark at gunpoint. Duncan directed Shasta to bind Brenda, Slade and Mark Mackensie with nylon zip ties. Then Duncan placed duct tape around their necks and placed the duct tape gags in each victim's mouth.

Duncan had the keys to Dan and Lisa Miller's pickup. He bound Shasta and Dylan and placed them in the pickup. Then he took a large hammer, went back into the house and bludgeoned the three bound victims. Afterwards, he drove the children to a side road near the Hollingsworth residence where the Jeep Cherokee was parked. He transferred them to the Jeep, abandoned the pickup and drove for several hours to a remote Forest Service campsite in the Lolo National Forest near St. Regis, Montana. Duncan bragged to the children about bludgeoning Brenda and Slade Groene and Mark Mackenzie. He repeatedly beat and sexually molested the children during the seven weeks they were held hostage.

He videotaped the abuse and his unspeakable acts before finally bludgeoning and shooting Dylan Groene to death. He attempted to dispose of the bones in a campfire and later discarded the body in a culvert a short distance away from the campsite. Duncan and Shasta Groene left the campsite on July 1, 2005 and drove back to Idaho.

Surveillance video from a Kellogg, Idaho convenience store earlier on July 1 showed Shasta examining goods on the shelves before leaving with Duncan. A convenience store owner recalled Duncan purchasing gas, a *carton of Bud Lite and asking for information about camping sites in the Lolo National Forest.*

*I am not aware whether Duncan bought additional supplies in St. Regis or another Montana town during the seven weeks he held the children in captivity.*

*The arrest of Joseph Duncan and safe recovery of Shasta Groene brought a sigh of relief to Coeur d'Alene and North Idaho. However, it also confirmed Dylan Groene's murder at the Montana campsite.*

*During the booking process, the extent of Duncan's criminal past came to light like an avalanche of horrors. A partial list of his rap sheet includes a twenty-year sentence for assaulting a boy in Tacoma, Washington, in 1980. After a parole in 1994, he was arrested again in 1997 for parole violation. He has also confessed to but had not been charged with the murders of two girls in Seattle in 1996.*

*At the time of his arrest in Coeur d'Alene, Duncan was driving the Jeep Cherokee, which he had rented in Minnesota. It had been reported as stolen when the rental period expired. He had jumped a $15,000 bail bond on a charge of assaulting a Detroit Lakes, Minnesota girl. Joseph Crary, a Fargo, North Dakota, businessman—provided the bail money. The Washington state parole board had denied his request to live at the home of Dr. Richard Wacksman, a pediatrician in Fargo, because children lived in the home. Dr. Wacksman provided Duncan with $6,500 prior to his leaving the Fargo-Moorhead-area enroute to Idaho. Analysis of Duncan's fingerprints linked him to the murder of a child in Riverside, California.*

*With the assistance of information derived from interviews with Shasta Groene, Detective Maskell traveled to St. Regis, Montana and located the campsite in the Lolo National Forest, where they found partially incinerated remains. DNA results from a small fragment of skull determined the body to be that of Dylan Groene.*

*An initial hypothesis that another person(s) contributed to this crime streak was never confirmed. Authorities concluded that only Duncan had committed the crimes.*

*After numerous delays, pretrial motions, and other defense maneuvers, a trial was scheduled in District Court in Coeur d'Alene. On the day the trial was scheduled to begin, Duncan entered a plea of guilty to three counts of murder and kidnapping of the Wolf Lodge victims. The Prosecuting Attorney, William Douglas, and the Public Defender, John Adams, indicated they accepted the plea to spare Shasta the ordeal of facing her kidnapper/rapist and family's murderer in court.*

*The District Court Judge sentenced Duncan to three consecutive life sentences without possibility of parole. Kootenai authorities withheld charging him with the kidnapping of Shasta and Dylan, pending the outcome of the federal trial for kidnapping, sexual torture, murder and transport across state lines, which are federal offenses.*

*During the subsequent federal trial, held in Boise, Idaho, Duncan argued with his defense attorneys, finally firing them, stating he wanted to represent himself. The U.S. District Court Judge, Edward D. Lodge, ordered a psychological examination to determine if Duncan was mentally competent to make such decision, and able to represent himself. Based on the examination of the three psychologists, the Judge Lodge determined that Duncan could represent himself and was competent to stand trial on the federal charges. The three defense attorneys, including Judy Clarke, a prominent capital defense attorney, remained as "standby counsel" during the trial. The jury found Joseph E. Duncan, III, guilty on all charges. US District Judge Edward Lodge sentenced Duncan to death by injection. Duncan gave up his right to appeal the decision. He was transported to the federal prison in Terra Haute, Indiana to await execution.*

*Meanwhile, Riverside, California authorities formally charged Duncan for the murder of **Anthony Martinez**. They transported Duncan from Terre Haute, Indiana back to Riverside, California, where he was tried and convicted of that murder, and given an additional life sentence. Detective Brad Maskell attended that trial, as well, to provide additional testimony against Duncan.*

*In 2013, seven years after the murders in Wolf Lodge, the Ninth US Circuit Court of Appeals remanded the case back to the US District Court in Boise, Idaho, for a "retrospective competency hearing." The Appeals Court's premise was that the competency hearing should have been held in open court rather than in the judge's chambers. Attorney Judy Clarke testified that she and the other defense attorneys did not realize the extent of Duncan's mental problems. Clarke said Duncan told the attorneys that, as he was about to bash Shasta's head with a rock, he had an "epiphany" and decided to let her live. He believed he was a "Jesus-like" figure for the world. Clarke said the risk of the death penalty did not much concern him.*

*On December 6, 2013, US District Court Judge Lodge issued a decision that Joseph Duncan WAS competent to make the decision to represent himself at trial, and that Duncan had rationally relinquished his rights to appeal. Joseph Duncan, III, is back in Terre Haute, Indiana, awaiting execution.*

As such, we are approaching the "average" duration for death penalty cases. It is likely that further appeals will be filed despite the ruling above. The Terre Haute Federal prison holds ninety-eight inmates on death row. Only three executions, including the Oklahoma City Bomber Timothy McVeigh, have occurred at the Terre Haute federal prison in the past ten years.

The Kootenai County Commissioners established a special billing account for the Duncan case. In 2011 at the last accounting, it exceeded $230,000 for Kootenai County alone. In addition, the ongoing costs of his incarceration approach $50,000/year. This illustrates the strain on personnel and resources these cases present. From the Coroner's point of view, it demonstrates why investigation and attention to detail can be crucial to ensure proper carriage of justice. As one detective in this case remarked to me, "It is up to the Good Lord to make judgement on Joseph E. Duncan, III. Our job is to make sure he keeps his appointment."

The "take-away" lessons from the Duncan case are myriad. It will be dissected for years for the lessons learned. Following are some issues we have discussed in various debriefing sessions:

## General and "Pre-Kootenai County" Issues

1. The criminal justice system, which allowed this chronic, repeat offender and sexual predator out on probation in the first place.
2. I am not aware of the terms of his probation from Washington State. However, when the Washington State Parole Board learned

of his re-location to the Fargo-Moorhead area, some mechanism should have kicked in to more closely follow his activities there.

3. Duncan attended college-level, computer and photography classes and acquired several digital cameras, recording devices, and computers during his sojourn in Fargo, ND.

4. The Washington State Parole board should have been alerted when Duncan traveled to the St. Louis area and then returned to Fargo.

5. When Duncan was arrested for the assault of the young man in Detroit Lakes, MN, queries to the National Crime Information Center (NCIC) should have produced his Washington criminal record.

6. The complicity or gullibility of:
    A) The Fargo businessman who wrote a $15,000 check for Duncan's bail on the assault charge; and
    B) The Fargo pediatrician who queried the Washington State Parole Board to have Duncan stay at his home even though there were children residing at the home, and then provided $6,500 "travel cash" for Duncan.

7. The car-rental agency that rented the Jeep Cherokee to Duncan and then did *not* initiate an alert when the vehicle was not returned on time.

Note: The automated license reading equipment had not yet been installed on I-90 at the Washington/Idaho border.

## Kootenai County Issues:

1. Amber Alert activation was slower and more cumbersome than we would have liked.

2. Prompt activation of the Command Center under the Office of Emergency Management.

3. Assembly of Multiple Agency team for briefing, prior to accessing and processing the Wolf Lodge scene.

4.  Enlisting FBI, regional and national agencies to complement local resources.
5.  Perimeter security and provision of shelter for the investigative team.
6.  DNA sample processing at the FBI lab in Quantico, Va., on an expedited basis. (DNA results on all of the bloody prints in the hallway and kitchen belonged to Slade Groene.)
7.  Fingerprints yielded only family member prints. Note: Duncan wore gloves while holding the family at gunpoint. He had Shasta apply the zip ties to the victims.
8.  Determination of the origin of the VCR movie "Taking Lives." Was it rented, and by whom? Was the cassette/slip case examined for prints?
9.  Utilization of single-source Public Information Officer (PIO) to issue all press releases.
10. Intensive use of missing person photo flyers locally and nationally.
11. Enlisting the public to supply tips, sightings, and other information.
12. Was Duncan identified as a "person of interest" prior to his arrest at Denny's? (Answer: No!)

## Court Proceedings:

### Idaho First District Court:

1.  Evidence and procedural processes were meticulous.
2.  Separation of the Wolf Lodge murders and kidnapping of Brenda and Slade Groene and Mark Mackensie (Idaho District Court) from the Federal Crimes of Interstate kidnappings, and the physical and sexual molestation of Shasta and Dylan Groene and the murder of Dylan Groene (Federal Court).
3.  Forensic autopsy findings prepared for presentation by the Forensic Pathologist from the Spokane Medical Examiner Office.

4. District Court accepted Duncan's guilty plea to all of the Idaho District Court charges on the day before the trial commenced.

## US District Court Proceedings:

1. The Federal Trial in the First U. S. Federal Court in Boise was complicated by Duncan's dismissal of the provided defense counsel, and acting as his own attorney.
2. The psychologic determination of Duncan's mental status and his ability to provide for his defense was decided by Judge Lodge in his chambers rather than in open court.
3. Duncan's relinquishment of a Right to Appeal of the Federal death sentence.
4. The Ninth Circuit Court of Appeals' order for "Retrospective Competency Determination."
5. Ruling by First Judicial U.S District Court on December 7, 2013, which found Duncan competent provide his defense and to act as his own attorney.

## Comment:

This case consumed multiple agencies for seven horrible weeks in 2005. The case is ongoing and appeals are pending. The above items are only listed as discussion points. I am not competent to offer comments on the legalities of various Idaho and Federal proceedings. I can state, however, that the evidence strongly suggests that Joseph E. Duncan III is a highly intelligent, calculating, career criminal. The degree of planning and execution (sic) of the many crimes he committed in Idaho and Montana is extraordinary. I have not reviewed the several psychological evaluations done during either Federal trial.

Fortunately, I have not had any direct contact with Joseph Duncan.

There are several encrypted files on the laptop computer seized from Duncan that local computer experts have been unable to open. Duncan has indicated in at least one of his appeals that he would offer to unlock the encrypted files as a bargaining chip.

Shasta Groene is an incredible young person. She used her innate survival skills to get her through her seven-week ordeal. She continues to make her recovery and recently returned to Coeur d'Alene. It is my non-professional opinion that Duncan brought her back to Coeur d'Alene as his "trophy" hostage, rather than the so-called "epiphany" he experienced in Montana. Whether she developed a 'Stockholm Syndrome' or not, is not my call to make.

Finally, I am impressed and thankful for all the effort expended by hundreds of people, both professionals and lay people. The public was well served by the various agencies during the dogged pursuit of this perpetrator of one of the most heinous crimes in Idaho history. I also know, from my perspective as Coroner, it is another example of the importance of collaborative efforts between the coroner and many other agencies. We each bring our unique orientation to every case. It is vitally important that we do not impede the work of other agencies. Mutual respect can go a long way to ensure a smooth operation.

Despite the entire scope of evidence gathering—DNA, fingerprints autopsies, etc.—it was a waitress at Denny's Restaurant at two o'clock in the morning who recognized Shasta, called the police and brought this nightmare to an end. For that we can be eternally grateful.

With the concurrence of all parties, the Groene residence was demolished and the area returned to its wetland status. However, none of us who were involved in this case can drive by Wolf Lodge without having memories flood back.

CHAPTER 19

# MASS FATALITY MANAGEMENT AND PLANNING

We have participated in local/regional Mass Disaster Plan development. Most readers will have been acquainted with similar activities or have been involved with disaster drills. All too often, such plans are finalized, and then relegated to some obscure file cabinet, only to be dusted off when an actual event occurs. Following the events of 9/11/2001, numerous Federal and State directives were promulgated to upgrade Mass Disaster Plans and Contingency for Mass Fatality Management.

It is interesting that some "knee-jerk" responses consisted of ordering hundreds of body bags to be stored in some warehouse, thinking that would take care of the planning! In actuality, detailed disaster plans have been developed to cope with real or hypothetical events. Some Northwest examples follow:

## The Sunshine Mine Disaster, 1972

The Sunshine Mine is a deep, hard-rock silver mine located about eight miles east of Kellogg, ID. Miles of tunnels service the workings as low as 4,100 feet below the surface.

*On May 2, 1972, one hundred seventy-three miners were lowered into the mine via the hoist over the Jewell shaft. About half past eight in the morning, a fire broke out deep in the mine, spreading toxic smoke and gases throughout the miles of tunnels. Some miners survived using their carbon monoxide absorbing masks. Eighty-three were rescued on May 2, two were rescued a week later. Ninety-one miners perished in one of the worst mining disasters in US History.*

*Kootenai Medical Center and the Kootenai County Coroner's office were placed on disaster alert. However, it soon became apparent that recovery efforts would involve retrieval of the bodies of the miners. Most of the miners had succumbed to high levels of carbon monoxide in the mine. Survivors told of many heroic deeds by miners in the depths of the mine, only to be overcome by the gas. Funeral homes from around the area sent morticians to assist Silver Valley mortuaries process and care for the deceased miners and console their families.*

A memorial monument to the miners is alongside Interstate 90 near Kellogg Idaho.

While the Kootenai County Coroner did not participate in the recovery and processing of the bodies, it was an object lesson on how quickly a disaster can overwhelm the resources of a community.

## Skydiving Accident near Yakima, WA

*A fixed-wing aircraft carrying nine skydivers and a pilot crashed in the Cascade Mountains near Yakima, Washington. When Search and Rescue teams recovered the remains, the bodies and body parts were brought to the King County Medical Examiner's office in Seattle. Reports from the King County Medical Examiner's office told of massive efforts to process the forty-plus body bags to make identification, issue death certificates, and release the remains to next of kin. These activities so overwhelmed the office they had difficulty keeping up with the steady flow of their regular cases.*

My point is that a metropolitan medical examiner's office was overwhelmed with the workload of nine fatalities, in addition to their "regular" caseload. It is entirely likely that a similar mass casualty disaster in North Idaho would overload the medical and coroner resources in Kootenai County, and to a lesser extent, Spokane County.

We have worked with the Panhandle Health District Region I, and Kootenai County, to develop a Regional Disaster Management Plan. We have Mutual Aid agreements with the coroners in the five northern counties to provide assistance in the event of a natural or man-made disaster.

Under the Robert T. Stafford Disaster Relief and Emergency Assistance Act, the Federal Emergency Management Agency (FEMA) has developed a unified approach for the delivery of mass care services by collaborative planning and pooling of resources. We developed a Mass Fatalities Response Framework document to provide an Emergency Morgue Facility at the USFS Tree Nursery in Coeur d'Alene. This facility has several climate controlled cold storage units, which could be utilized as an Emergency Morgue Facility. The Tree Nursery has a single, secure access point and the capability to handle mass fatality victims while not disrupting its primary mission. The nearby Salvation Army Kroc Center has been identified as a family service location.

When the Governor (and/or the President) declares a "Disaster Emergency," several federal agencies may be activated under the umbrella of the Federal Emergency Management Agency (FEMA.) These include:

- Disaster Mortuary Operational Response Teams (DMORT)
- Disaster Portable Morgue Unit (DPMU)
- FEMA, Department of Defense (DOD)
- National Transportation Safety Board (NTSB.)

It is important to remember that all of the above must be done under a "Declared Disaster Emergency" for the local agencies to be reimbursed under FEMA.

DMORT and DPMU provide personnel and equipment to fully implement an emergency morgue. Local personnel would have to cope for up to seventy-two hours while the equipment is transported from a regional depot in Oakland, California to Kootenai County. DMORT personnel also need to be mobilized and travel to Coeur d'alene.

As with all such plans, however, a real or simulated disaster drill will undoubtedly uncover various deficiencies and corrections will be made. The Spokane County Medical Examiner's office has reviewed and supports the North Idaho Regional Disaster Plan.

## The Great Greyhound Bus Caper – February 1981

*One of the more bizarre law enforcement episodes in North Idaho occurred in February 1981. A Greyhound bus traveling from Missoula, Montana, to Spokane, Washington, stopped in Wallace, Idaho, at about ten o'clock in the evening. The driver, Charlie Justus, removed a disruptive, inebriated passenger with mental problems from the bus, and continued west on Interstate 90.*

*The inebriated, unruly passenger went to the Wallace Police Department and reported an armed hijacker had taken control of the bus and its nineteen passengers. Police radios broadcast warnings of a potential hijacking-hostage situation. We were notified of the ongoing chase and awaited for further updates.*

*By the time the bus pulled into the Greyhound bus stop in Coeur d'Alene, a convoy of unmarked and marked patrol vehicles from the Idaho State Police, Kootenai County Sheriff and Coeur d'Alene Police were tailing the bus.*

*Not wanting to force an armed standoff in the urban environment, the officers allowed the bus to proceed on I-90 toward Spokane. Two Idaho State Police Drug Task Force officers, dressed as scruffy hippies in an unmarked Chevy Malibu, responded to the purported hostage/hijacking. The order was given to stop the bus. The Malibu pulled alongside the bus, waving the driver to pull over and stop.*

*The bus driver, seeing two "hippies" waving him over, now was certain he was being hijacked. Finally, the convoy boxed the bus in and stopped the bus.*

*The undercover ISP officers, shotguns in hand, jumped out of the Malibu and ordered the driver to surrender. The bus driver, seeing this "hippy" aiming a shotgun aimed at him, dove for cover. As the bus lurched forward, the ISP Officer shot out its two front tires, and another deputy shot out the two rear tires. Justus and nineteen shaken passengers exited the bus with arms raised, uncertain of their fate.*

*Finally, the hoax was sorted out after further questioning of the original passenger. The passengers were transferred to another bus brought over from Spokane. Greyhound paid for the destroyed tires, and ISP paid for the damages to the bus. Of course, the media had a heyday to the discomfiture of all concerned.[12]*

This "disaster that wasn't" was another example of the planning necessary to deal with such events. The need to confirm the reported hijacking and collaboration of multiple agencies in the middle of the night is paramount. The restraint of officers in not causing bodily harm to the bus passengers, driver, or to each other is to be commended.

---

[12] Clark, Doug, "The Man who shot a Greyhound Bus, February 1981," Spokesman-Review, 2006. (Used by Permission.

# CHAPTER 20

# GUNS, AMMO AND THE SECOND AMENDMENT

I cannot calculate what percentage of the estimated 300 million US firearms are located in Kootenai County. In Idaho, the Second Amendment is practically an article of faith. In addition, NRA membership is substantial. In the course of responding to numerous coroner cases over forty years, I am continually amazed at the number and variety of weapons in Kootenai County. Nevertheless, the majority of the weapons are rifles and shotguns used in hunting. I have personally seen almost every known caliber and model of gun produced in the world in these collections. The weapons range from derringers, dueling pistols, "elephant" guns, AR-15s to Thompson submachine guns, and even an authentic US Army artillery piece produced to specifications in US Army Ordnance blueprints.

One collection numbered over a thousand guns, some of which had never been fired. Others were weathered and worn from hunting trips and exposure to the elements of outdoor Idaho. Likewise, gun owners maintain more than adequate supplies of ammunition for their weapons. The CCI ammunition plant in Lewiston, Idaho, provides ammunition in a wide variety of calibers and loads, even muzzleloader rifles. The Ponsness-Warren plant in Rathdrum manufactures ammunition-loading equipment for the general public. The Cabelas store in Post Falls carries an extensive line of supplies for home loaders including smokeless and black powder, cartridges and bullets in a myriad of calibers and weights. Numerous other retail outlets in Kootenai County and neighboring Spokane, Washington have an abundance of new and used weapons.

Not *all* citizens in Idaho belong to the National Rifle Association (NRA.) A member of the NRA National Board of Directors lives in Coeur d'Alene. A high percentage of Idahoans, male and female, are gun owners and a smaller percentage of them actually hunt.

Gun safety courses are mandatory for young hunters and would be desirable for adults as well. Indoor and outdoor ranges are popular venues for instruction and maintenance of shooting skills. The number of concealed-carry weapon permits skyrocketed after 9/11. New applications continue at a brisk pace.

*I responded to a home in Coeur d'Alene where a man had used a lever-action Winchester .30-30 carbine to commit suicide. In the basement of the home, there were more than twenty such rifles in near-mint condition. This model, first produced by the Winchester Firearms Company in 1894, is considered one of the classic rifles of the American West. A footstool, made out of an elephant's foot, stood at the base of the stairs as well as numerous other trophies adorning the walls attesting to the hunter's prowess.*

*In another instance, I was called to the residence of a nurse I had known while on staff at Kootenai Medical Center. I would characterize her as a very competent nurse, with a passive and unassuming demeanor. She was a devout Mormon. The basement contained the requisite year's supply of non-perishable food in various plastic, five-gallon containers. All were labeled as to contents, date of purchase and rotation dates.*

*The most notable thing about the house was that there were numerous, loaded guns about the house. A loaded 12-gauge shotgun was standing behind the front door; another rifle was in the living room, as well as the suicide weapon found next to the victim. This lady was the most unlikely person to possess such a collection of weapons.*

*One of the challenges which law enforcement faces, in such cases, is to carefully inventory and disarm such weapons without endangering themselves or others on scene.*

*I responded to a suicide incident at a Coeur d'Alene iron foundry. The owner had used a large-caliber revolver to self-inflict a fatal head wound. At the time of my arrival on scene, KCSO officers had secured the weapon. The owner's wife stated that when her husband became increasingly depressed over financial and other matters, they had removed a 38 cal. revolver from the office. Deputies had been unable to locate the second weapon in the office. With her permission, we made a detailed search of the premises as well as their residence, to no avail. At last, I made a careful pat-down search of the victim and found the gun secreted in his trousers!*

I have always been exceedingly careful not to send any bodies to the SCME office without first making absolutely certain any weapons are on the victim.

*In one Bonner County case, a revolver dropped out of the body bag just as the pathologist was preparing to do the autopsy. "Not a good way to foster good relations with your local medical examiner."*

Efforts at gun control in the wake of several mass shootings have been largely futile. This is partly a result of a strong gun lobby (especially the NRA), and partly widespread support of the Second Amendment. More effective mental health programs are needed to identify those persons with violent tendencies, or who will not take medications to control their symptoms. As more and more psychiatric patients are treated on an outpatient basis, there is an increased likelihood that mentally ill people will be in the community and may present problems with firearms.

There are 50 percent fewer in-patient psychiatric beds in the United States than we had at the time of passage of the Firearms Control Act in the Kennedy Administration. With an estimated 300 million guns in the United States, it is unlikely that gun control measures will seriously diminish that number. Background checks and an efficient, accessible database would help prevent unauthorized persons from obtaining weapons.

Note: Joseph Duncan, a convicted felon, (Chapter 18) had no difficulty in obtaining the gun he used to hold the Groene family at gunpoint before bludgeoning them to death.

Over the years, I have developed a deep respect for gun owners. There are many areas in the county that I will not enter without the escort of an armed law enforcement person.

*A Kootenai Electric Co-op crew called me to investigate an electrocution in Cougar Gulch. The lineman had come in contact with the grounding wire as the pole was being set in the post-hole. The crew had encountered a very hostile property owner who ordered them off his property at gunpoint. They had to discontinue line maintenance at his property line, and advised me not to go beyond the stricken lineman. Naturally, I followed their directions.*

# CHAPTER 21

# DRUGS, METH LABS AND OTHER HAZ-MAT SITUATIONS

Alcohol remains the "drug of choice" for abusers in Idaho, as it is in the rest of the country. The subject of alcoholism, treatment, and lethal hazards are well known and go beyond the scope of this book.

Kootenai County is somewhat unique in our location astride a major North-South Highway (US 95) and Interstate 90 going East-West. We are only thirty miles from all of the urban drug problems of Spokane, Washington. Mixed messages are being sent with the recent legalization of the sale of marijuana in the State of Washington. In addition, the shift from state liquor stores to liquor sales in large grocery outlets despite a substantial tax on the sales has had a dual effect: 1) the profitability of small liquor stores in Washington has made their financial survival questionable. 2) Buyers now travel to Idaho for liquor that is cheaper and does not have the higher taxes.

The drug pipeline from Mexican drug cartels supplies dealers with an abundant supply of drugs to supply to Kootenai users. "Mules" hauling backpack loads of British Columbia weed ("BC GOLD") across our porous northern border keep the narcotic task force on constant alert. Recently, the use of unmanned drone-type aircraft to patrol several hundred miles of the US-Canadian border has augmented agents on the ground.

High-grade methamphetamine and cocaine show up regularly in our coroner cases. We get toxicology on many cases and with a high percentage of mixed drug overdoses. Having toxicology gives us a 'canary in the coal mine' alert to the varying spectrum of drugs in the community.

Recipes for methamphetamine production abound on the Internet and in the drug underground. I am always astounded at the ability of a high-school dropout to acquire the basic chemicals and equipment for meth production. The toxic red phosphorus and volatile solvents contaminate such sites.

*We discovered one such clandestine lab in a rental house in Hauser Lake. A decomposing body had phosgene (mustard gas) in the toxicology done by the SCME. Blood spatters appeared around the house, but most of the equipment had been removed. One trailer load of glassware and chemicals was intercepted in Montana, southbound to Salt Lake City, Utah. Another vehicle was found heading for the Tri-cities in Central Washington.*

The cleanup of these labs frequently consumes more time and money than the building is worth. Haz-Mat workers take extreme precautions not to trigger explosions from ether and other solvents used in the process. Toxic red phosphorus and volatile solvents further contaminate such sites. It behooves coroners to exercise care while investigating these sites.

Heroin arrives from the poppy fields in Afghanistan by way of an extensive smuggling network that stretches across Asia to the West Coast. Our eleven-plus years in Afghanistan have done little to dissuade poppy farmers to plant other cash crops. Nationally and statewide, there is a rise in heroin cases and with several fatalities involving heroin admixed with fentanyl. So prevalent is the problem that many poison control experts have suggested that paramedics carry pre-loaded syringes of Narcan in their drug kits. Narcan combats the respiratory depressive effects of Heroin/Fentanyl.

*I responded to a reported 'knifing' victim in Coeur d'Alene. The police officer escorted me to an adult male found in the bathroom of the apartment with multiple linear, superficial lacerations on his back. I determined the "lacerations" were actually the result from his cat scratching the lifeless body.*

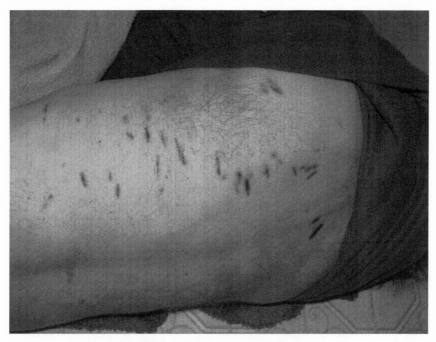

"Cat Scratches on Heroin Overdose Victim"

*When we autopsied the body, however, the toxicology showed an unsuspected heroin overdose. He had no local relatives. However, interviews with his psychologist uncovered his drug habit.*

*A veterinary technician from Montana was found deceased in a local motel from an overdose of the anesthetic drug, Propofol. It is a powerful sedative with rapid onset, used during induction of anesthesia. It is also highly addictive and subject to abuse, as in the recent Michael Jackson case. The technician had diverted several syringes loaded with the drug from the animal hospital where he worked. We found several expended cartridges of the drug in wastebaskets in the motel room.*

High-grade methamphetamine and cocaine show up regularly in coroner cases. We also get toxicology reports showing a high percentage of mixed drug overdoses. Using advanced toxicology labs gives us a 'canary in the coal mine' alert to the varying spectrum of drugs in the community. Coroners must be aware when new drugs appear on the illicit drug market.

The recent appearance of the street drug "Molly" a highly refined, crystalline form of MDMA, the active ingredient in the drug 'Ecstasy,' is one example. It is one of a group of "designer drugs" making the rounds of rock concerts and other gatherings. Others include: '2-CP', 'Butane Hash Oil'- (used in "dabbing".) Onset of symptoms may take as long as ten hours before the victim becomes unconscious. Butane explosions during the distillation process have become fairly common. 'Krokodil,' a derivative of codeine mixed with oil, gasoline or other solvents and injected in the skin, leaves a leathery scaly scar, hence the name. It is important that coroners/medical examiners be aware of the presence of these illicit drugs in the local population and be alert for the side effects and residual signs. Once again: It Can and Does Happen Here!

# CHAPTER 22

# UNIQUE ASPECTS OF TEENAGERS

No *one* term can describe the wonderful world of the teenager. One day they are a pimple-faced child in a developing body. The next, they are serious young adults ready to face the world with all of its problems. One parent I know describes them as "a bundle of hormones and sex on wheels." Perhaps the term "bullet-proof" typifies their mentality. The incredible potential of their intellect and energy continues to amaze me, as well as their parents. An in-depth discussion of the teenager must defer to another time.

Raising five children in Kootenai County through their elementary, high school and college years and interacting with other teenagers does _not_ make me an expert on such matters. It does give one a perspective on the emotional and physical development they experience. The raw emotions they experience when one of their own is killed in a car accident or commits suicide is painful to watch.

No parent is immune to the anxiety when Junior takes that first solo car ride or when the first prom night is looming on the weekend. Yes, there are occasional heartbreaks when a late night party ends up in the ditch with dreams shattered forever. Despite their outward bravado, they are really fragile, developing individuals. We need to nurture them in many ways to avoid producing a wounded psyche or a broken body. This process starts in the cradle and lasts well past their emergence into adulthood. 'Letting go' is almost as hard as raising them but somehow they manage to survive and go on to bigger and better things. I have been careful to maintain the privacy of coroner cases. There have been times when a ride-along has served as an object lesson to the realities of life and the inevitability of death.

It is important that coroners be aware of the hazards to which teens are exposed and develop strategies to deal with them. Alerting parents to signs of underlying psychiatric problems, especially depression can offer an opportunity to intervene prior to rash actions.

Peer group pressure accounts for some of the alcohol and drug use in teenagers. Access to liquor at home, or from adults who purchase and provide it to teens, is a major problem. "Keggers" held in remote areas of the National Forest lead to teens driving home drunk. Many fatal accidents occur on winding treacherous forest roads. A significant number of these drivers and passengers are not wearing seatbelts, which increases the likelihood of ejection from the vehicle and higher fatality rates.

Intervention and prevention may come from a variety of sources. However, much more needs to be done to prevent this intolerable waste of lives, talent and resources. The recent resurgence of heroin overdoses is of concern to all coroners and is cause for additional toxicology testing.

The desensitization resulting from violent TV, movies, and video games may blur a teen's sense of reality. There is a ready source of drugs available in unlocked home medicine cabinets. Pain pills such as Hydrocodone (Vicodin), Oxycontin (Percodan) and other psychoactive drugs are more often obtained from these sources than from street vendors.

The flawed prescribing habits of some physicians result in prescriptions for addictive narcotics when non-steroidal analgesics or other analgesics would suffice for pain control. When a teenager is given a refillable prescription for sixty Oxycontin for an ankle sprain, the stage is set for a developing addict.

Adults need to be aware of some of the unusual behaviors exhibited in cases I have witnessed. "Huffing" of the propellants in pressurized cans of vegetable or hair spray in a plastic bag can result in a hypoxic death in a very short time. The propellant displaces oxygen in the lungs and the victim suffocates. We have had cases of autoerotic gratification by breathing in a plastic bag resulting in asphyxiation.

A more serious type of behavior is the so-called "Choking Game." It also goes by such names as: "Pass out Game," "Scarf Game" or "Space Monkey." Pressure is applied manually, or by means of a noose, by the victim or another person, directly to the carotid arteries, shutting off circulation to the brain. This causes brief cerebral hypoxia and unconsciousness. The victims report a surge of euphoria or erotic stimulation upon release of the pressure. However, cardiac arrhythmias or serious neurologic effects and some deaths may result from the practice. Such deaths may result in homicide charges being filed against the participants. The CDC's Morbidity, Mortality Weekly Report (MMWR) of February 2008[13] reported eighty-two deaths in youths, ages six to nineteen, between the years of 1995 and 2007. There are no CDC guidelines for reporting these deaths and many are classified as suicides due to self-strangulation.

Typically, the teens will not self-report the behavior until a tragedy results. Parents, health professionals, coroners and medical examiners need to be aware of the existence of this syndrome.

A national awareness Web site, www.gasp.org, provides more information. Parents and educators need to be aware of some of the physical signs such as petechial hemorrhages on eyelids, neck bruising and headaches—and seek early intervention. Opening the conversation is at least as difficult as teenage sexual counseling, but stands to reap many benefits for the teens and society.

---

[13]    Morbidity & Mortality Weekly Report (MMWR) CDC, February 2008

# CHAPTER 23

# DEATHS IN CUSTODY

## Jail Deaths and Deaths in Custody

Inmates get sick like the rest of the population. Jail deaths, however, get extra scrutiny because of the nature of the population. Suicides occur despite precautions taken during incarceration. Individuals will fashion ligatures out of bed sheets, towels, or other items. Often the victim has been cut down and/or taken to hospital and we are faced with re-constructing the crime scene. It is challenging to gather the all facts from jail personnel who may have been our co-workers on other cases. We almost always autopsy such deaths to determine whether an underlying medical condition or trauma was responsible for the death.

## Inmate-on-Inmate Violence

Although the presence of prison gangs rare in the county jail setting, the occurrence of such violence and deaths must be carefully investigated to identify perpetrators and separate them from the rest of the jail population.

## Drug Deaths

We have investigated several cases in which drugs have been smuggled into the jail and ingested with fatal consequences. More common are cases where an inmate suffers a fatal overdose from drugs ingested prior to incarceration. The combination of alcohol and drugs can represent a lethal situation.

## TASER® Deaths

(NOTE: Taser® is a registered trademark of Taser International. All rights reserved.)

Tasers® were developed by Jack Cover, a NASA engineer in the 1960s and 1970s. It is an acronym for Tom A. Swift Electric Rifle, named after a comic hero in the twentieth century. It is classified as an Electronic Control Device (ECD.)

First deployed in 1998, some 514,000 of the weapons are in use by law enforcement and the military around the world. A civilian model is also available. There has been some controversy over their use with some suggesting they should be classified as "near-lethal" rather than "non-lethal." The United Nations Commission on Torture (UNCAT) report of 2007 listed the Taser® as a "form of torture."

The TASER® Model X26 fires two darts connected by wires to the weapon. It delivers a 5,000-volt, 1-amp discharge, which immobilizes the victim and allows law enforcers to apply restraints. It can also be used as a contact device.

A 2001–2007 summary of 245 deaths following Taser use listed the cause of death as "could not rule out (r/o) Taser as the cause of death."

In September 2007, a twenty-one-year-old University of Florida student, Andrew Meyer got in a scuffle with police. His plea: "Don't Tase me, bro!"™ was listed as the quote of the year by the *Yale Book of Quotations.*

TASER® International has been very vigilant against any implications that Taser-related deaths be classified as a homicide. A fifty-six-year-old, wheelchair-bound, female victim died after being Tasered in 2006. The Coroner listed the manner of death as a homicide. TASER International sued the Coroner and won a judgment. The District Court judge ordered the death certificate to be revised to, "cannot r/o cause of death due to Taser" and the manner of death as "accidental."

Nonetheless, the consent form[14] required for all Taser® course students and instructors covers two pages, and includes a specific liability release and covenant not to sue Taser International or the instructor. The form lists a litany of physiologic or metabolic effects, which may result from Taser® use. These include, but are not limited to, changes in blood pressure, and heart rate and rhythm, which may increase or cause death or serious injury.

Most arrest-related deaths (ARD) occur in agitated states due to concomitant drug and/or alcohol, or because a victim is otherwise compromised. Taser use in cases of "excited delirium" has an increased incidence of ARD.

We have investigated several cases classified as "excited delirium" where the victims were either high on cocaine or methamphetamine. I am not aware of any deaths in Kootenai County in which Taser® use was a factor.

---

[14]  Taser International, "Instructor and User Warnings, Risks, Liability Release and covenant Not to Sue" Taser International, May 2011

# CHAPTER 24

# INTERNATIONAL RELATIONS – COEUR D'ALENE INDIAN TRIBAL MATTERS

The Coeur d'Alene Indian Tribe is a sovereign tribal nation which lies within portions of Kootenai and Benewah Counties. It also includes the lower one-third of Coeur d'Alene Lake. The Kootenai County Coroner investigates all deaths on the reservation from 'other than natural causes.' These may also involve the Coeur d'Alene Tribal Police, the Bureau of Indian Affairs, the FBI, Kootenai County Sheriff department and the Idaho State Patrol.

The Tribe has developed a large Casino, Hotel and Golf Course complex just north of Worley, Idaho on the reservation. Increased traffic resulted in the construction of a new bypass on U.S. 95. The revenues generated by these entities have been distributed to regional schools and colleges, as well as the construction of a well-staffed health facility at Plummer, Idaho and a variety of other endeavors.

The Tribe has a fireworks display annually on the Fourth of July. A storage unit contained the fireworks for the display as well as two propane tanks and other miscellaneous items. Two tribal members were working in the unit when an explosion occurred involving the fireworks and the propane tanks and resulted in the deaths of both tribal members.

Our investigation involved multiple agencies including the EPA, OSHA, and members of the units above including the Kootenai coroner. Because of the industrial implications and our investigation, both bodies were autopsied. No illicit substances were found on toxicology.

*     *     *

One stormy January night, I received a call from a KCSO Deputy who had been called to the Casino for an unattended death. His first words to me were: "Doc, I just spent two hours navigating a nearly closed Highway 95 in my four-wheel drive SUV. I have an unattended death here but I would advise you not to try and respond."

He related the following history:

A Kellogg couple had driven to Worley via Route 97 which is a winding 2-lane highway. At the time, the weather was snowing and windy but otherwise passable. The wife had undergone open heart 5-vessel bypass at a Spokane hospital in the remote past. She had developed a worsening, ischemic cardiomyopathy and was in progressive cardiac failure. As a last-ditch effort, her cardiac surgeon had implanted a battery powered left ventricular assist device to bridge her until a suitable heart for transplant became available. She was a long-time smoker and was on multiple cardiac medications. After checking into the hotel, they spent a considerable amount of time playing the slot machines in the casino.

As they were having dinner at the restaurant, she noted that the low-battery alarm on her portable pack was sounding. She excused herself and went up to her hotel room to change the batteries. When she did not return after an hour and a half, the husband went up to the room and found her deceased on the bed, holding the connecting battery cable in one hand and the connection port to the device in her other hand.

I elected not to attempt to respond to the Casino due to weather and road conditions on the advice of the KCSO Deputy. I think that was the only time that I failed to respond to a coroner call.

One cannot help but wonder at the wisdom of the couple to brave an Idaho blizzard to travel to a gaming casino or the husband's lack of concern for his wife to get the vital battery change process. The medical decision to implant an experimental device in a non-compliant patient raises concerns as well.

I did recover the assist device when her body was brought to a Coeur d'Alene funeral home and had it shipped to the manufacturer in Massachusetts to determine if there had been any malfunction.

# CHAPTER 25

# ORGAN AND TISSUE DONATION

In 1954, Drs. Joseph E. Murray and John H. Harrison, in collaboration with nephrologist Dr. John P. Merrill, performed the world's first successful kidney transplant between identical twin brothers at the Peter Bent Brigham Hospital in Boston, Massachusetts. Because identical twins share the same genetic material, there was no rejection of the transplanted kidney.

Lectures by Dr. Murray to my medical classmates at Harvard were exciting as the whole field of transplantation expanded. Immunosuppressant drugs like Imuran and Cyclosporine prevented rejection problems in transplants between unrelated individuals. By 1970, kidney, heart, lung and pancreas transplants had been successfully carried out in the United States and around the world. Dr. Murray received the Nobel Prize in Medicine in 1990 for his work in the development of transplantation procedures.

*In the early 1970s, I was the on-call surgeon when a young man was brought to Kootenai Medical Center with a severe head injury and numerous other injuries. The unconscious victim had fixed dilated pupils and signs of brain herniation. It was apparent the head injury was non-survivable. The young man's father, a neurologist from Spokane, arrived at the hospital. We informed him of the extent of the brain injury and the likelihood that he would not survive. The father asked if his son could be an organ donor. We concurred that he was an ideal candidate for organ donation. Arrangements were made for his kidneys to be harvested at the time of his demise. His kidneys were harvested at another hospital and transplanted into two recipients successfully.*

The subsequent rapid expansion of organ transplantation resulted in the National Organ Transplantation Act of 1984. The act prohibited the sale of organs, formed a national database for organ sharing, and developed a registry of organ recipients scaled by relative urgency for transplant, and locations of the donor and patient. Kootenai Medical Center participated by developing local protocols for use in "brain dead" patients, developing a relationship with regional organ procurement agencies, and encouraging patients to become organ donors. Strict bioethical guidelines are followed to ensure that all necessary care is given to the patient until a diagnosis of "brain death" has been documented under nationally accepted criteria.

Under the 1984 Transplant Act, all hospital and physician charges following the declaration of brain death are paid for by the Organ Procurement Organization (OPO) at no cost to the family. The attending physicians for the patient are not allowed to participate in organ recovery.

Families and hospitals receive follow-up from the OPO as to location and course of the recipients. Identities of the donor and recipients are always kept anonymous.

I was active in implementing these protocols and also took training courses to recover kidneys at Oregon Health Sciences University in Portland. We have had several donors who met criteria for heart-lung, liver and kidney donations with successful transplantations of the organs in multiple recipients.

It is a rewarding experience to see an unmitigated tragedy transformed into a life-saving new lease on life for the recipients. The Organ Procurement Coordinator is required to obtain consent from the Coroner prior to commencement of the organ retrieval. Coroner consent for post-mortem harvest of corneas, skin, and long bones is also required.

Organ donation has never resulted in criminal charges against a perpetrator being dropped. Extensive testing of donors to assure tissue matching, blood typing, HIV status, rabies, hepatitis, and others are all part of the OPO protocol. (Note: A corneal transplant recipient in Southern Idaho developed a fatal case of rabies when an undetected rabid bat bite had occurred prior to the donor's final illness.)

Public forums to encourage people to register as an organ donor are routine. Each Idaho driver licensee renewal is asked whether he/she wants to be an organ donor. It is important that donors inform family members of their decision to avoid some of the conflicts arising when a potential donor has not informed the family.

As of this writing, there are more than 121,000 persons on the national organ transplant waiting list. Each day, several of the 2,000 patients on the Pacific Northwest waiting list die for lack of a donor. Between January and September 2013, 21,659 transplants were performed in the United States. Of those, 17,265 were from deceased donors and 4,394 were from living donors. Note: Many organ donations result in multiple recipients.

It behooves coroners and medical examiners to educate themselves on the subject and facilitate the process of donation as a part of their responsibility to the public. Life Center Northwest is the regional Organ Procurement Organization (OPO). The reader is referred to the United Network for Organ Sharing Web site at www.unos.org, or Life Center Northwest at www.lcnw.org.

# AFTERWORD

# WHERE DO WE GO FROM HERE?

It has not been my intent to depict Idaho as a hotbed of death and destruction. Rather, I hope that by relating some of my activities for more than four decades as Coroner in Kootenai County we can begin a serious discussion about improvements in the coroner/medical examiner system. It is likely that many similar vignettes occur in any city or county in this country. The Public deserves a better system than we have at present. We can only get a better system if the public becomes better informed as to the actual situation at hand, and takes whatever action required towards improving the system. Certainly, coroners in many jurisdictions do a great job under difficult circumstances. Greater personal responsibility to educate oneself as new diagnostic problems and challenges arise. The worst enemy is complacency- "Nothing ever happens around here" or "We just cannot afford to autopsy another case or incur huge bills for toxicology testing." are familiar refrains to nearly every coroner/medical examiner.

It is not likely that many of the deficiencies of the present death investigation system can be resolved overnight. However, several suggestions follow:

1.  Educate yourself on the coroner/medical examiner system where you live. What are the educational qualifications and certifications of the people holding the office?

2.  Insist on adequate funding for the coroner/medical examiner in your state or county. To simply declare or to legislate a State or County Medical Examiner System without funding or adequate planning assures an even more dysfunctional system than we already have.

3.  Ensure that there is close collaboration between *all* of the various entities: law enforcement, coroner/medical examiner, funeral homes, hospitals and medical staff. Territorial prerogatives, voluntary inertia or bureaucratic obfuscation contribute to dysfunction in this area.

4.  Encourage more health professionals to become involved in death investigation, including physicians and other healthcare workers. Expansion of pathology and forensic pathology training programs to help reduce the ~1,500-person shortage of medical examiners in the United States.

5.  Address many of the "fixable" items listed in this book including: suicide prevention programs, drunk driving prevention, alcohol and drug prevention, seat belt usage and marine safety education.

6.  Look in the mirror! Do any of the situations outlined pertain to you or your loved ones?

7.  Discuss Organ Donation, Tissue Recovery, and Durable Power of Attorney for Medical Care with your family.

8.  Remember: "It Can and Does Happen Here!"

# ABBREVIATIONS

AMI – Acute Myocardial Infarction
ATV – All Terrain Vehicles
A.W. – Atomic Weight
BNSF – Burlington Northern, Santa Fe Railroad
CAD – Coronary Atherosclerosis
Cda PD – Coeur d'Alene Police Department
CDC – Centers for Disease Control
CFS – Cubic Feet per Second
COPD – Chronic Obstructive Pulmonary Disease
CVA – Cerebrovascular Accident
DPMU – Disaster Portable Mortuary Unit
DMORT _- Disaster Mobilization and Recovery Team
DNA – Deoxyribonucleic Acid
ECD – Electronic Control Device (see Taser)
EPA – Environmental Protection Agency
FAA – Federal Aviation Administration
FBI - Federal Bureau of Investigation
FEMA – Federal Emergency Management Administration
ISP – Idaho State Police
KCSO- Kootenai County Sheriff Office
KMC- Kootenai Medical Center-(now Kootenai Health)
LCNW – LifeCenter Northwest - (An OPO)
PFPD – Post Falls Police Department
NAMUS – National Missing and Unidentified Persons System
MI - Myocardial Infarction (Also called AMI)

MMWR – Morbidity, Mortality Weekly Report (CDC)

NCIC – National Crime Information Center

NRA – National Rifle Association

NTSB – National Transportation and Safety Board

OPO – Organ Procurement Organization

PTSD – Post Traumatic Stress Disorder

PTSS – Post Traumatic Stress Syndrome

SCME – Spokane County Medical Examiner
         (Forensic Institute)

SHMC – Sacred Heart Medical Center, Spokane, WA

TASER™ – Tom A. Swift Electronic Rifle

TIA – Transient Ischemic Attack

UNOS – United Network for Organ Sharing

USAF – United States Air Force

USFS – United States Forest Service

# BIBLIOGRAPHY

"Charles Norris (1868-1935) and Thomas A. Gonzales (1878-1956,) New York's Forensic Pioneers" American Journal of Forensic Medical Pathology 1987 Dec 8 (4) pp 350-353

Clark, Doug, "The Man Who Shot a Greyhound Bus, February, 1981" Spokesman-Review, 2006

Eckert, W.G., *"Medico legal Investigation in New York City. History and Activities 1918-1978," Am.* J Forensic Med Pathology, 1983, Mar: 4 (1): pp33-54

Flowers, Eric, "Charges Filed in Benway Case," Coeur d'Alene Press, Feb 1, 2001 (Used by Permission)

Idaho Code: Chapter 31, Sec. 2801-2807 (Coroner To Act as Sheriff); Chapter 34, Sec. 6422 (Qualifications for Coroner)

Joiner, T.J. *"Myths about Suicide"* Harvard University Press 2010

Kershner, Jim, *"Pulaski's Legacy Alive in Standard Fire Tool,"* Spokesman-Review, August 17, 2010

Knox, K.L., Litts, D.A., Talcott, G.W., Feig, J.C. Caine, E.D.2003: *Risk of suicide and related adverse outcomes after exposure to a suicide prevention programme in the U.S. Air Force: cohort study:* British Medical Journal, 13,327, (7428)

Kristof, Nicholas and WuDunn, Sheryl, *"Half the Sky," Alfred E. Knopf, New York, 2009*

McLain, Mike, "Benway's Mother thankful" Coeur d'Alene Press, Feb 1, 2001. (Used by permission)

Morbidity & Mortality Weekly Report (MMWR), CDC, February 2008

Quinette, Paul, *"QPR– Question, Persuade, Refer" www.QuinetteInstitute.com*

*"Smoking and Health: Report of the Advisory Committee to the Surgeon General"* CDC 1964

*"Reducing Suicide: A National Imperative"* National Academies Press, 2012

*"Settlements Being Readied for Some Downwinders"* Environmental Defense Institute, Volume 21, Number 8, December 2010

*Strengthening Forensic Science in the United States"* National Academies Press, 2009

*"Sudden Unexplained Infant Death"(SUID),* Centers for Disease Control and Prevention(CDC), August 2013

Taser International, *"Instructor and User Warnings, Risks, Liability Release and Covenant Not to Sue"* Taser International, May 31, 2011

# Acknowledgements

The events in this book have been gleaned from Kootenai County Coroner records, Court Transcripts and my own recollection of the incidents. The *Coeur d'Alene Press* and *Spokesman-Review* have given permission to quote from copyrighted materials in published news reports.

I owe a debt of gratitude to my wife, Martha, who has been my mainstay of support. She rode "shotgun" on many of my midnight forays into the backwoods of Kootenai County. Fortunately, her numerous knitting projects occupied her time while waiting for me to complete a death investigation. Our five children, Steve, Chris, Anna, Cathy, and Sarah provided the impetus to record the events which occupied so much of my time over forty years as Deputy Coroner and Coroner.

Thanks, also, to my deputy coroners: Jody Deluca-Hissong, LPN; John Hunt; Richard Halligan; Debbie Wilkey, RN, MA; and Lynette Acebedo, CNA. My office staff including Candace White; Judy Thormahlen; Janet Funk, RN, Judy Bliven, RN, Patsy Sorenson, RN and Kay Magruder, RN managed to reschedule patients, answer many phone calls and complete thousands of forms and letters in the course of my tenure.

Thanks to members of the law enforcement community -- Kootenai County Sheriff, Idaho State Police, Coeur d'Alene Police, Post Falls Police, and Coeur d'Alene Tribal Police -- as well as surrounding communities. The professional respect and collaboration we have shown for each other has made this project enjoyable and useful to the public.

Special thanks to the Spokane Medical Examiner's Office for providing forensic services of outstanding caliber and professionalism.

The mutual collaboration and communication between our offices has been a pleasure.

The services and personnel of Yates Funeral Homes, English Funeral Chapels, Belltower Funeral Home as well as the funeral homes of surrounding counties have greatly assisted the Coroner to carry out his duties. I could not have done this without your constant assistance and professional services.

Lastly, I want to thank the people of Kootenai County who entrusted me with the privilege of serving as your Coroner. May we all strive to learn from the experiences in this book and to seek improve the Coroner/Medical Examiner system in Idaho and the United States.

My editors, Ann N. Videan and Donna Bonham West have provided guidance and helped steer me toward the road to grammatical correctness. To all the folks at Abbott Press, I want to express my appreciation for their help in bringing this project to fruition.

\*    \*    \*

# ABOUT THE AUTHOR

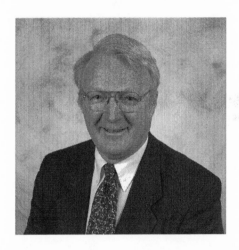

Born on a farm in southwestern North Dakota, Dr. Robert West spent seven years as a part-time "Printer's Devil" during high school and college. He did his premedical studies and the first two years of medical school at the University of North Dakota. He transferred to Harvard Medical School, receiving his M.D. degree in 1961. Following five years in the Medical Corps of the United States Navy, Dr. West completed a surgical residency at the University of Vermont Medical Center Hospitals. Dr. West, Martha, and their five children moved to Coeur d'Alene, Idaho, in 1969.

He served on the surgical staff of Kootenai Medical Center for thirty-four years, retiring in 2003. He served as a deputy coroner from 1970 until being elected as Kootenai County Coroner in 1984 to 2011. He oversaw the institution of advanced emergency and paramedic pre-hospital care and provision of full-time emergency physicians. Dr.

West provided coroner coverage for the 1,441 square miles of Kootenai County as its population soared to 130,000 people.

The mix and complexities of coroner cases have multiplied over the years and provided the cases described in this book. His wife and children provided the impetus to record the cases and be an advocate for change in the Coroner/Medical Examiner System in the United States.

Dr. West served his community as president of the Idaho Medical Association and the Idaho Chapter of the American College of Surgeons, and the Coeur d'Alene District #271 School Board.

For twenty-five years he played baritone horn in the zany Perfection-Nots band in the Fourth of July parade in Coeur d'Alene.

Since retiring as Coroner in 2011, he and Martha spend time visiting their children, twelve grandchildren, and three great-grandchildren, as well as pursuing his hobbies of beekeeping, boating on Lake Coeur d'Alene and Puget Sound, and traveling.

He maintains his interest in improving coroner issues of continuing education, qualifications, and funding for death investigation.

\*     \*     \*